THE HEALING DIET

THE HEALING DIET

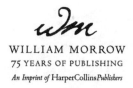

A Total Health Program to
Purify Your Lymph System and
Reduce the Risk of Heart Disease,
Arthritis, and Cancer

GERALD M. LEMOLE, M.D.

WILLIAM MORROW
75 YEARS OF PUBLISHING
An Imprint of HarperCollins*Publishers*

Portions of Chapters 6 and 10 were originally published in 2000 in *An Integrative Approach to Cardiac Care* by Gerald M. Lemole, M.D., and Medtronic, Inc.

HarperCollins books may be purchased for educational, business, or sales promotional use. For information please write: Special Markets Department, HarperCollins Publishers Inc., 10 East 53rd Street, New York, NY 10022.

FIRST EDITION

Designed by Kate Nichols
Medical, massage, and exercise drawings by Pat Stewart
Graphics courtesy of Medtronic/Lemole

Library of Congress Cataloging-in-Publication Data
Lemole, Gerald M.
    The healing diet : a total health program to purify your lymph system and reduce the risk of heart disease, arthritis, and cancer / by Gerald M. Lemole.—1st ed.
        p.   cm.
    Includes index.
    ISBN 0-688-17073-0
    1. Heart—Diseases—Diet therapy.   2. Heart—Diseases—Prevention.   3. Lymphatics.   I. Title.
RC684.D5 L46   2001
616.1'20654—dc21   00-038306

01   02   03   04   05 QW 10   9   8   7   6   5   4   3   2   1

To my wife, Emily Jane,

with admiration, respect, and love

Contents

Acknowledgments

I would like to thank Richard Marek without whose literary ability this book would not have been written. I'd also like to thank Ivan Kronenfeld, Carl Koerner, and Mitch Douglas for introducing Richard to the project. Last, I would like to thank Eileen McKiernan, Nancy Lafferty, Nanci Catinella, Lynne Smith, and Doris Odhner who were so invaluable in producing the manuscript.

THE HEALING DIET

Introduction

On the day I began to write this book, I performed three heart bypass operations. Two were scheduled in advance, both of them relatively easy cases. The third was an emergency. A woman with a history of previous heart problems, in the hospital for a stress test, had suddenly suffered a full-blown attack and needed to be operated on immediately. I had planned to start the book in the afternoon; now it would have to wait until night.

I tell you this to show you how routine it all is—I have performed or directed more than 20,000 heart surgeries, most of them without complications, and no major problems developed during any of the operations that day. Even emergency operations like the one described above, although often more perilous than operations prepared for in advance, are hardly uncommon. It would have been riskier when I first started thirty-three years ago, and it always amazes me to see how far we've come in such a short period of time.

Today quadruple bypass operations—even heart transplants— are simply taken for granted. Hundreds of doctors—not just a handful—are now well qualified to perform them. In nonemergency cases, some 98 percent of the patients survive; only when it's an emergency does the figure go down to 92 percent. In hospitals all over the world, people's lives are being saved because we've built new routes in the body for blood to reach the heart, or installed a machine to keep a heart pumping, or substituted one heart for another—and no one, with the possible exception of the patients and their loved ones, thinks that anything particularly out of the ordinary has occurred. They *expect* us to save lives. That's what cardiac surgeons are for.

I wouldn't have begun contemplating the ordinariness of cardiac surgery were it not for the fact that I have an important story to tell. But now, when I reflect back on the day, two important concepts, which I've been pondering for years, coalesce:

1. Thirty years ago, what I did so ordinarily today would have seemed like a miracle.
2. Far fewer heart attacks, far fewer emergency operations, and far less need for cardiac surgeons would exist if people took care of their lymphatic systems.

•   •   •

For as long as I can remember, I wanted to be a doctor. My father owned a pharmacy on Staten Island, and he, my mother, my two brothers, and I lived in an apartment above it. Quite naturally, doctors were among my father's closest friends, and several of them played in his weekly card games. My favorite, Bob Calta, was a surgeon. He had four daughters and no sons, and he took a special interest in me. He had played minor league baseball, and since I was an avid athlete and played high school baseball, basketball, and semipro football we had a special bond. The stories he told of his work, of dramatic cuttings and tumors extracted in the nick of time, caught and held my imagination. In those days surgery was far less sophisticated than it is now. The surgeon had fewer advanced technological tools at his disposal and was more reliant on his own technical skills and good judgment.

Maybe part of my enthusiasm came from my heritage. Somehow the potentially volatile combination of an Irish mother and an Italian father worked to my benefit. I can be sharp and incisive if I see someone about to make a mistake. I like to test the mettle of my team when things are going well, to see how they'll later respond to an emergency, but in a crisis I am calm and in control. Whatever the genetic factor, it works well in the OR.

I was a premed major at Villanova and went on to Temple University Medical School. After an internship at Staten Island Hospital, I returned for a surgical residency to Temple, then as now one of the great hospitals in the country.

Through it all I wanted to be a general surgeon, but at Temple Hospital I began hearing of the transplant surgery that was being performed in Houston, and this new procedure—this "miracle"—excited me so much that I became determined to make transplantation a specialty. To do so, of course, general surgery was a first essential, so I continued my residency.

In 1963 Dr. Michael DeBakey, who headed the surgical program at Houston, came to lecture at Temple. He talked not only of artificial hearts but of the possibility of transplanting *human* hearts. I asked the dean at Temple to recommend me to DeBakey for a position there. Happily for me, he did so gladly.

So in 1967, at the age of thirty, I arrived in Houston to learn hands-on a brand-new methodology—and I loved it.

It's difficult to describe how thrilling those few years were. We were all virtual novices in as yet undertested techniques. Yet we were doing coronary bypasses and heart transplants—one at a time, slowly, often clumsily—and we were often successful. We didn't know much about immunology. We didn't fully understand why one heart would beat and another wouldn't. Why, we asked ourselves, would an electrocardiogram show an increased heart rate in the patient when the heart beneath our fingers was beating no faster? To see a person on an operating table, chest open, heart removed, and then to put another one in—this was pretty exciting stuff. We would often spend weeks with our patients while they recovered (or, in some instances, died). We would sleep in their rooms, spending twelve hours on call for them, twelve off. Still, I was rarely tired. I felt I was in the world's most advanced physiology lab. I was learning a new science from brilliant pioneers.

I worked not only under DeBakey, who was by then concentrating on lung transplants (talk about miracles!), but also alongside Denton Cooley, codirector of the program. He was experimenting with artificial hearts. My colleagues and I were truly astronauts of science, walking on terrain no one else had explored.

•   •   •

The rest of my professional history was relatively straightforward. The heart became the abiding interest of my professional life. I decided to concentrate not only on transplants and bypass surgery but on operations that were often simpler though no less life-giving. Because we were having trouble with the transplants: too frequently the patients' bodies rejected them, and in those cases, of course, there was no hope for their survival, I wanted to find ways to make the operations safer and more reliable.

In 1969 I returned to Philadelphia and became an instructor in surgery and soon thereafter chief of cardiothoracic surgery at Temple. In that same year, I performed the first coronary bypass in the tristate area of Pennsylvania, New Jersey, and Delaware. Three years later, while keeping my post at Temple, I became chief of surgery at Deborah Heart and Lung Center in Browns Mills, New Jersey, and at the age of thirty-eight became a full professor at Temple, one of the youngest ever in the United States.

In 1986 I was asked to become head of the cardiac surgery division of the Medical Center of Delaware (now named Christiana Care Health System), a job I've held ever since. Not the least of the reasons for my satisfaction there is that thanks in part to the generosity of the Du Pont company and family, the center is superbly equipped; another is that it's a marvelous training facility for younger surgeons; and a third is that the staff that surrounds us is as good as in any hospital I've ever seen. You can't perform cardiac surgery without teamwork. At the center, we are a smoothly functioning team.

I consider myself a good scientist, a surgeon who has mastered both his craft and the medical machines that have made it easier. I am very much a part of the "medical establishment."

But along the way, several things happened to broaden my scope. Now I view surgery and its attendant equipment—lasers, endoscopic instruments, heart-lung resuscitators—as only one part of the cure for heart disease. I have become as interested in prevention as I am in cure. I'm aware that diet, exercise, lack of stress, and abundance of spirituality (yes, spirituality) are essential for a sound heart. And I'm also aware of the part the lymphatic system plays, not only in determining a well or ailing heart but in cancer, arthritis, and many other chronic diseases as well.

• • •

The first of the events that broadened my view took place at Temple soon after I returned from my stint at Baylor—after, remember, a number of our heart patients had crashed.

A senior pathologist named Betty Lautsche, whose specialty was the function of foam cells (you'll learn what these are later on), noticed a striking number of cases of accelerated atherosclerosis in heart transplant patients. She wondered whether the cutting of the lymphatics—an unavoidable consequence of the transplant operation—might be responsible for increased blockage.

As chief of cardiac surgery, I collaborated with other departments in research projects. Betty asked me to operate on some rhesus monkeys to see if I could confirm her theory that interruption of the lymphatic system in her heart patients was responsible for the transplants' "galloping" atherosclerosis. If that's the case, I thought, perhaps other enemies of the lymphatics—obstruction caused by cholesterol, shallow breathing, lack of exercise, and/or release of the adrenal hormones cortisone and epinephrine—could cause the hardening of arteries. So I agreed to perform the operations.

After interrupting the lymphatics of the monkeys' hearts, I fed them a diet high in cholesterol for several weeks. *All of them developed severe atherosclerosis.*

It took no great leap of the imagination for me to figure out that if we could rid the human body of high cholesterol and other toxins by cleansing the lymphatic system, we would go a long way toward preventing atherosclerosis. As far as I know I was the first to have recognized this. I was excited by the new idea, and I vowed to investigate it further.

Shortly thereafter I attended an international conference in Austria. At this symposium the effects of cholesterol were discussed. In its unoxidized form, cholesterol is manufactured by the liver and acts as the basic building block of the cell walls. Scientists had found that cholesterol moves in and out of the cell membranes thousands of times a second; it is, quite simply, essential to life. However, when it is oxidized, it is an extreme irritant to the cell walls.

Since cholesterol is a fatlike substance, it doesn't dissolve in water, so to be transported and delivered to the cells through the bloodstream, it must be joined to a lipoprotein. You can think of the added lipoprotein as a kind of mailbag. By using radioactive tracing, the researchers were able to see that the cholesterol carried by low-density lipoproteins (LDL, sometimes called "bad cholesterol") stopped at the elastic membrane of the artery wall. High-density lipoproteins (HDL, or "good cholesterol"), on the other hand, carried the cholesterol through the artery walls into the lymphatics, and from there eventually to the liver, where it can be metabolized—broken down into its components—along with other toxins. The cholesterol carried to the cells by low-density lipoproteins is metabolized at the *tissue* level, leaving the cholesterol free. This "pure" cholesterol is a substance used by the body for repairing damage; as I said, we cannot live without it. But often there is a residue. Ideally, high-density lipoproteins pick up any excess material not used in repair and carry it through the lymphatics to the veins and then on into the liver.

But things do not always work the way they should. Atherosclerosis, for example, is itself a damage the body is trying to repair. The problem is that it can be *over*repaired—too much cholesterol brought to the rescue, so to speak—causing a narrowing of the blood vessels and thus, among other things, impeded blood flow to the heart.

The place where lipoproteins carry cholesterol along, clearing it from the cells and carrying it through the heart to the liver, is the lymphatic system. Thus it became apparent to me that *the way to a healthy heart is through the lymphatics*. Patently, if we could keep the lymphatics—the body's cleansing system—clear, the cholesterol would travel easily, and little or no cholesterol would build up in the arteries. The arteries would remain unclogged, and the heart would receive enough blood to allow it to beat normally.

There was no question that the lymph system had to remain clean. The question was how?

•   •   •

One answer, I came to realize, was through diet.

When I was a freshman in medical school, I met a beautiful woman named Emily Jane Asplundh, then in her first year of college. We went out a few times but soon separated. I was a traditional Roman Catholic, she a Swedenborgian, and our theological arguments—one in particular about the nature of evil—were what I most remember about those first dates. When we met again three years later, we began dating seriously. Seven months later we were married.

After I started my residency, Janie began going through my medical journals, clipping out articles she thought would interest me. In effect, the process introduced her to medicine, and gradually she expanded her reading—and clipping—to books and newspaper and magazine articles about the healing power of foods and herbs. Later her reading focused on the healing effects of stress management and spirituality. This was long before the concept of mind-body medicine had reached the American consciousness, and I was definitely one of the skeptical scientists who discounted most of it.

But I didn't discount Janie's ideas. She wasn't a kook or a flower child. I knew her spirituality came from a deep faith and commitment to God, her focus on diet from what became years of study in the area of nutrition and holistic health. But while I trusted her intuition, I thought she was uneducated in science and medicine.

"You don't understand what doctors *do*," I said.

"Doctors don't have *training* in health, diet, and nutrition," she answered.

Doctors are taught pharmacological medicine, Janie pointed out. Americans go to doctors and say, "Help me. Give me a pill to feel better." The prescription is a quick fix—the American way.

But too often it's the wrong approach. It concentrates on elimination of the symptoms, not the cause.

"The hard work of changing lifestyle and diet can make an enormous change in people's lives," Janie recently told a newspaper reporter. "It isn't a substitute for medicine. It *complements* medicine. Much of being healthy is a choice."

I had to agree with her. In my four years at medical school, and throughout my residency, I could count the number of lectures on nutrition on one hand. Their focus was on "a well-balanced diet," but such a traditionally well-balanced diet was in fact a myth.

My conversion to Janie's way of thinking came slowly. But when the connection between diet and the lymphatics was made clear, I thought I'd try Janie's regimen on my heart patients. Maybe vitamins and herbs, vegetables and fruits would help clear the lymphatic system. Maybe the risk of a second heart attack could be reduced.

So even twenty years ago, while the medical establishment scoffed at the "health food fad" endorsed by, among others, Adele Davis and Nathan Pritikin, I began to put my patients on a low-fat, high-vitamin diet. "They'll never get back their strength," doctors told me. "You'll kill them." They threatened to stop referring bypass candidates to me. By then, fortunately, I had achieved a good enough reputation as a surgeon that the patients themselves insisted on seeing me; anyway, my practice didn't suffer. (Ten years previously, the medical establishment had believed that if patients exercised after a heart attack, they would surely die, a philosophy now also discredited.)

My patients didn't suffer either. Indeed, they found that a vegetarian diet did wonders for the heart. My patients got better faster and had fewer relapses. In every area of their health they became vital, younger-seeming, *well*.

Sometimes, even when it's too dangerous to perform heart surgery, patients can be helped by diet. For example, recently a woman named Cheryl came to me in desperation after two New York heart surgeons had told her that her failing heart had so damaged her liver that her body could not tolerate surgery. They were right: the operation *was* impossible unless her liver failure was reversed. But how could she reverse it unless her heart was repaired?

Janie suggested that Cheryl be put on a regimen that included very high doses of vitamin C and an herb called milk thistle. I felt it was her only chance. Since Cheryl knew something about herbal medicines, she believed me and went home to follow the program.

Six weeks later, when she came back to the hospital, blood tests showed nearly perfect liver function. She was then able to undergo the heart surgery. She is alive and healthy today, getting a degree in social work so she can express her gratitude for having gotten a second chance.

Please don't misunderstand me. I am a firm believer in conventional medicine; I've seen its miracles. Heart transplants and bypass surgery are the culmination of hundreds of years of continual medical advances, including the growing sophistication of machines and the invention of the laser. In the next hundred years, genetic engineering will have so progressed that we'll be able to eliminate congenital heart disease before a baby is born as well as to eradicate other genetic diseases, such as sickle-cell anemia and Tay-Sachs disease.

Traditional medicine and holistic approaches can complement each other and optimally be integrated into the very best plan for the individual patient. I am absolutely convinced that "alternative medicine" is *medicine,* and to ignore its effects is to be blind to an important ally in health care. Indeed, better terms than *alternative medicine* are *complementary medicine* or *integrative medicine.* To forsake one form of therapeutics and rely wholly on the other as the only way to health is to ignore evidence gathered over thousands of years that nature and science are twin soldiers in the fight against disease.

And when it comes to *prevention*: well, there I am a proselytizer for holistic regimens, as ardent and committed as my wife.

•   •   •

This book is primarily about disease prevention. If you have heart malfunctions, you may need heart surgery; if you have cancer, you may need surgery to further treatment. But if you keep your lymphatic system clear—*and I promise you can do it naturally*—you can eliminate 70 percent of the chronic illnesses that are in part the result of that system being clogged.

As an introductory step, you must first be *aware* that chronic disease is caused by defective lymphatics. If I could take you into the operating room with me and show you the deposits of cholesterol on the arterial walls of the heart—cholesterol left there because LDL deposited it and there was not enough HDL to carry it back into the lymphatics and on to the liver, where it could have been metabolized—you too would swear off butter, meat, ice cream, and chocolate fudge in a second.

But you can't come with me and can't see what I see on a daily basis, so all I can do is take you through the program I've designed for myself and others. It isn't radical, it isn't painful, it won't make you abnormally skinny (although you won't be fat), but it *will* keep you in optimal health for the rest of your natural life.

First of all, I exercise. And the major exercise I do is breathe.

I'm not talking about the unconscious breathing that all of us do every moment of our lives. Rather, I'm referring to deep, *conscious* breathing. The air pressure in your chest drops so that your lungs can work like a bellows, exercising the area around the heart. When you inhale, the air pressure in your chest drops down, sucking lymph fluid along with it. Exhale, and the fluid is squeezed forward, the valves around the heart opening and closing as in any system of sluices. Remember, material carried by the lymphatic system travels through your chest on its way to the liver. Deep breathing speeds the process. It allows the lymphatic flow to course strongly and evenly, becoming virtually a river of life.

Notice that I said *deep* breathing. When we're anxious or afraid, we tend to take rapid, shallow breaths, and our heart rate must correspondingly accelerate. A little speedup is often beneficial (the heart needs its exercise like the rest of our body), but stress and fear, unlike exercise, stifle the breath and thus cramp the lymphatic system.

I recommend that you, too, take some time during the day to breathe deeply, inhaling and exhaling through your nostrils, feeling the breath not only in your chest but in your abdomen and diaphragm. Most books on holistic health separate breathing and exercise, but to me breathing is a form of exercise.

I also walk a mile or two each day, either outdoors or on a treadmill, or "rebound" on a trampoline. This is to get my heart rate up to about 120, again for the purpose of strengthening the heart and making sure the lymphatic system flows freely. I play golf and occasionally basketball, but otherwise I don't feel the need for more strenuous exercise. I admire people who swim, run, play tennis, and otherwise work up a sweat during the day. However, for the purposes of keeping the heart and the lymphatic system healthy, such exercise is not necessary, though it does benefit muscle tone and aids in weight loss. Correct exercise, not "big" exercise, is the key.

•   •   •

I don't eat meat. I did, up until eight years ago, but Janie convinced me to stop. Janie eats a basically vegetarian diet, though she includes fish occasionally. All of our six children have followed the same path except one, who still includes poultry.

Actually, I think human beings weren't really designed to eat meat. Unlike all carnivores, our teeth are not sharp; we can't tear meat from the bone the way a wolf does, and our back teeth are made for grinding, not cutting. Unlike a leopard's or a panther's intestines, which are short so that meat is quickly eliminated from the body, ours are long—28 feet long!—so the journey of food through our body is an arduous one.

According to evidence in the Bible, the earliest humans were primarily vegetarians. Meats were reserved for special days, and the Israelites were warned against the "fleshpots" of Egypt (*fleshpot* meaning exactly that: the Egyptians cooked meats in *ollas*—pots— adding more meat as the pots became depleted), for it was there that lust and overindulgence were rampant.

Meat is far more difficult to digest than vegetables. After not eating meat for years, I decided to have a small steak at a dinner party one evening, only to find that my digestive system, accustomed to more benign matter, could no longer handle it easily, and I was sick the next day. The fat in meats adds to the buildup of cholesterol and also delivers toxic chemicals (insecticides and antibiotics) and harmful hormones to our bodies. Soy or a variety of beans and grains supplies the necessary protein far better than flesh foods. And there are economic and ethical questions as well.

Later in this book I'm going to present you with a complete diet as part of a lifelong program for lymphatic health. My own diet now includes grains, soy, vegetables, fruits, beans, some fish, green tea instead of coffee, a glass of wine with dinner (one, not two), and vitamins and minerals at each meal. Janie, who has a master's degree in theology, is working toward a degree in nutrition and naturopathic medicine. It is her knowledge, far more than mine, that informs this part of my program.

Janie and I use a variety of herbs, garlic, olive and flaxseed oils (avoiding margarine and commonly available vegetable oils), soy sauce, and other natural flavorings. I like pepper but use minimal salt; I don't smoke (among other things, it's constricting to the lymphatic system); I drink six to eight glasses of water a day, and we eat out often, generally in Italian, Thai, or Japanese restaurants, where many of the dishes are vegetarian (for Janie) or fish (for me).

On all working days, Janie packs my lunch for me. Yesterday it was a cup of organic bean soup, a sheet of bran cracker, two organic carrots, some pink grapefruit sections, and a variety of vitamins and minerals. You might be able to have better-tasting food at Lutèce, but you won't find anything healthier.

•   •   •

Two other factors can keep your lymphatic system healthy: massage and stress reduction.

Sixty years ago, Dr. Theodore Drinker found that by massaging a dog's neck he could keep the animal's lymphatics flowing freely. The same holds true for humans.

In the next chapter you'll see diagrams of the lymphatic system. Massage in key areas will keep it toned, much as massage helps tone muscles. Besides professional massage, partners can massage each other. Simple, easily learned techniques will be illustrated in a later chapter, and many massage books and videos are now available. Massage is a powerful mover of lymph, and touch in itself is beneficial.

One reason the East German athletes did so well in the Olympic games of the 1970s and 1980s is that they were massaged before and after every event. This freed their muscles from tension, allowed all their systems, including the lymphatic, to regain full circulation, and removed lactic acid and other toxins from their tissues. Today most of our athletes receive similar massage treatments. On the professional tennis circuit, for example, Pete Sampras, among others, brings his personal masseur along with him.

As for stress reduction, it is so important that I'll devote more than one chapter to it in my description of the program. Stress, as any engineer will tell you, is the result of change, of two or more forces in opposition. Well, it's life changes that cause stress, not life's routines. All of us experience change; the goal is to react to it positively. It's not what happens to you from the *outside*. What matters is what happens *within* you.

People tell me that I must be leading a very stressful life since I perform as many as four heart operations a day. "Your patients' lives are literally in your hands," they say. "How can you not feel the pressure?" The answer is that heart surgery comes as easily to me as writing copy does to the copywriter or fixing a car does to the mechanic. Surgery for me is a creative blend of work and play. When you love what you do and do what you love well, you enter a different dimension. If I were forced to do something else—and particularly if I were forced to do nothing—*then* I'd feel stressed.

If you can *respond* to stress in a positive way, if you can substitute spirituality for anxiety, if you can fill your head with good thoughts and understand your anger and pain and know what to do with it, your lymphatics will prosper. Yes, the mind has a remarkable effect on lymphatic health.

Later I'll show you why. But it's time to turn to the lymphatic system itself, to show you more precisely how it works and exactly why it's so vital.

The Lymphatic System

Think of a forest pool. You have carefully built it into the mountainside just below your house. Fresh water from the top of the mountain pours into it whenever it rains or when the snow melts. At the bottom of the pool is a drain that, when opened, allows the water to flow out and continue on its way down the hill to the river at the bottom.

Perfect! Perhaps you even have such a pool. But even if you don't, surely you have a sink in your kitchen, which fills when you turn on the tap and close the drain, and empties when you open the drain and turn off the tap.

When as much water is coming in as can be emptied by the drain, everything flows smoothly. The pool remains fresh—ideal for swimming.

But what if the water carries with it silt and leaves and other refuse from the mountain. Sometimes the drain will get clogged, and the water will be unable to flow out. It will lie inertly in the pool. Then when new water comes, the pool will overflow, leaving

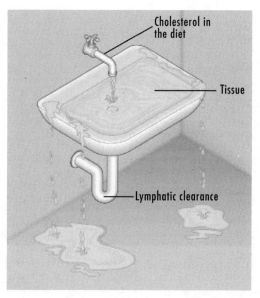

Cholesterol overload. Too much water in a small sink blocks the drain,
which is analogous to an inflammatory reaction in the vessel (tissue).

a residue of silt and leaves—and bacteria as well. The pool will
become fetid, unsafe for swimming.

The lymphatic system operates in much the same way. But
when it backs up, the consequences to your health are far more
serious: Heart disease. Arthritis. Cancer.

The lymphatic "pipes" are similar to those in the cardiovascular
system (the bloodstream) in being vessels that circulate the body's
fluids. The lymphatic system serves as the conduit through which
the lymphatic fluid (termed *interstitial fluid*) flows from around the
cells back into the blood system. Between the finest blood vessel,
the capillary, and the cell itself is located a sea of fluid, the lymph.
Across that sea oxygen and sugar are transported to nourish the
cell, and the cell's wastes—carbon dioxide, lactic acid, and metabolites—are carried back to the bloodstream.

Two kinds of pressure are involved: *hydrostatic pressure* (blood
pressure), which tends to force fluid out of the vascular system into

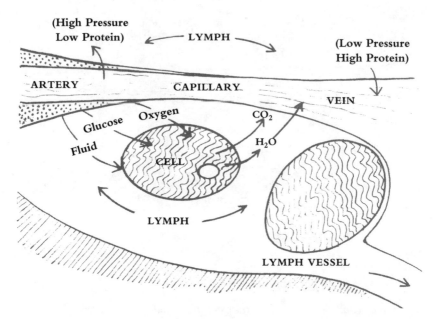

Diagram of lymph cell and vessel and the interactions with artery, capillary, and vein

the lymphatics; and the counterbalancing *oncotic pressure* exerted by blood proteins suspended in fluid.

For example, blood enters the capillary. The pressure of the heart muscle beating behind it forces its rich oxygen and sugar into the interstitial fluid. After the blood has passed through the capillary to the capillary's "downstream" end, it has lost some of its water in the process of nourishing the cell. Its proteins are therefore in thicker concentration. Now the blood takes on water from the interstitial fluid, which contains metabolites, carbon dioxide, and lactic acid, and continues on its way.

This marvelous mechanism not only offsets protein and pressure imbalances within the body but allows for clearance of potentially damaging elements.

Lymphatic pathways begin as tiny open-ended vessels similar to capillaries. These merge into larger vessels with walls similar to our veins. Like veins, they have flaplike valves that help prevent the backflow of fluid. The lymphatic vessels lead to specialized organs called *lymph nodes* (also known as lymph glands), located in the neck, the thoracic cavity (which contains the heart), the armpits, the abdomen, and the pelvis. These are the only parts of the system familiar to most people.

But too much emphasis has been put on the nodes, at the expense of the lymphatic system itself. Perhaps this is because swelling of the nodes is such a dramatic danger signal. Lymph nodes are not really conduits for lymphatic fluid but simply act as filters to remove particular threatening substances from the system. These include bacteria, viruses, and other foreign proteins, which are fairly large compared with oxidized cholesterol and other toxic substances that are the culprits in chronic diseases. Blood chemicals too small to be captured in the nodes must be metabolized by the liver and kidneys after being carried there by the lymphatics.

The nodes are like the water purifier you might use under your kitchen sink. Lymph nodes are the center for the production of *lymphocytes* (which act against foreign particles such as viruses and bacteria) and *macrophages* (which engulf and destroy foreign substances like damaged cells and other cellular debris).

Infections and diseases may be caused when microorganisms called *pathogens* enter the body. Diseases may also be caused by substances produced *within* the body, such as abnormal cells. When a virus, say, enters the body, it is seen as a foreign protein—an *antigen*. The body reacts by creating an *antibody* to destroy the perceived intruding protein. Substances as seemingly benign as tomatoes, peanuts, or chocolate can create antibody production and an allergic reaction.

The immune system, of which the lymphatics are an essential part, acts to fight off pathogens and antigens. It is, in essence, our own center for disease control, and we must keep it well funded.

*   *   *

After leaving the nodes, the lymph vessels merge to form still larger lymphatic trunks. These empty into the *thoracic duct*, which traverses the entire chest and opens at the bottom of the neck, just above the left collarbone, in what we call the supraclavicular space (in some people, a smaller thoracic duct is located on the right side of the chest cavity). Fluid in the thoracic duct is pumped along by the breath. A bellows mechanism, breathing exerts both a positive and a negative pressure. If you take a deep breath and exhale deeply, you're massaging the thoracic duct upward into the neck so that the fluid flows generously. This duct empties the lymph into the veins, where it becomes part of the blood's plasma. From there the lymph returns to the liver for metabolization, and finally to the kidneys for filtering.

Lymph, like blood, will not flow regularly or evenly without outside pressure. The blood has the heart muscle to pump it along; the lymphatics simply employ (less powerful) muscles nearby, including those of the skeleton, and the breathing to move lymph along. In both cases, flow is essential. Any severe disruption of either system will inevitably lead to disease or death.

*   *   *

In summary, flow of the lymph thus carries off chemicals along with whole and partially used up proteins and brings them back to the liver, where they are metabolized and excreted. Sometimes, as in the case of HDL, substances are reconstituted rather than excreted, so that they can be sent on a continuing journey through the body.

Unlike our other circulatory system, the blood, the lymphatic system is virtually unknown to the average person. Yet twice as much lymph as blood is present in your body, and twice as many lymph vessels as blood vessels.

The lymphatic system is as essential to bodily function as the bloodstream it complements. To keep it clear, you need to increase its drainage capacity or reduce its intake of toxins—and I suggest doing both.

For example, picture yourself in a helicopter flying over Eighth Avenue in New York City. Below, you can see that the avenue is filled with taxis, all going at a uniform speed. At Fortieth Street they exit the city, moving across the river to New Jersey through the Lincoln Tunnel; at Canal Street they come back through the Holland Tunnel and start uptown again. Every minute, ten cabs go through the Lincoln Tunnel and ten different cabs come back through the Holland Tunnel.

Now, what if we could widen the tunnels? Patently, the traffic would move more speedily; maybe you'd get twenty cabs going in either direction in that same minute. The taxis on the avenue would go faster; in case of an unexpected roadblock, there would be less congestion.

If you think of the two tunnels as the lymphatic system, Eighth Avenue as the bloodstream, and the yellow cabs as the HDL in which oxidized cholesterol "passengers" travel, the analogy becomes clear. (The LDL could also be visualized as cabs, only they drop their cholesterol passengers off where you don't want them to be left.) The purpose of this book is to help you widen your lymphatic system and thus make certain that more HDL cabs are available. Many otherwise enlightened people think that if they simply take an antioxidant, they ensure that their cholesterol won't become oxidized and they can safely go on eating as they have before. (To see the effects of oxidation, cut an apple in half and watch it turn brown. If you put vitamin C on it, this oxidation process won't occur.) But antioxidants, like any vitamin program by itself, are at best stopgaps, mops that will soon become hopelessly waterlogged.

Far better to adopt a complete program for the continuous cleansing of the lymphatic system. Through exercise, massage, diet, proper breathing, and stress modification, you'll free your lymphatics of unnecessary traffic and make space for more toxic cholesterol to be picked up by the HDL and carried away. This continuous-clearance program is the best solution for both prevention and treatment of disease.

·   ·   ·

Now, since I'm a cardiac surgeon, I want to emphasize how care of the lymph affects the heart.

In 1980, in a paper for the *Journal of Thoracic & Cardiovascular Surgery,* I postulated that slowing of the lymphatic system (technically, *lymphostasis*) is a critical factor in the genesis of atherosclerosis. Cardiac lymphatics had already been implicated in disturbances such as arrhythmias, bacterial endocarditis, and endocardial fibroelastosis. Now I was saying that inadequate lymphatic clearance of the arterial wall was a possible cause of atherosclerosis as well.

My thesis pulled together seemingly unrelated risk factors: the action of a pituitary hormone that constricts the smooth muscles of the lymphatics; personality; genetics, obesity and other aspects of family history; and simple aging. All these can have profound negative effects on the cardiac lymphatics. So can such factors as stress, cigarette smoking, hypertension, overeating, and inactivity. My paper also mentioned what is perhaps the greatest villain of all: cholesterol.

As noted, unoxidized cholesterol is essential to the lining of cell membranes and to brain tissue; we could not live without it. But *oxidized* cholesterol is one of the toxins carried—or not carried—by the lymphatics to the liver by way of the heart.

The lymphatic vessels leading to the arteries of the heart are divided into three layers: the *endocardial* (inner), *myocardial* (middle), and *subepicardial* (outer). Oxidized cholesterol is deposited only on the subepicardial artery wall. In the other places, cholesterol can be picked up by the HDL in the lymph and taken back into the blood. Obviously, the lymph cannot do this job once the proteins are stuck down and cannot be moved.

Within the lining of the heart artery, through which the vital tissue fluid flows, we also have three layers: the *intima* (innermost), *media* (middle), and *adventitia* (outer covering). The lymphatics of the heart artery collect the HDL from the adventitia. If a flush of HDL is not passing through the artery wall from the intima into the media and thus to the lymphatics, less of the oxidized cholesterol will be picked up. More oxidized cholesterol will be left in the intima, thus causing a toxic reaction.

The subepicardial lymphatics are just a series of channels. As exercise increases the force of contraction of the heart muscle, and deep breathing drops the pressure in the chest, lymph flows from the heart to the large collecting tube in the chest (the thoracic duct). The pressure that drives the flow from the deeper layers of heart muscle increases the pressure in the lymph channels on the heart's surface. This, plus the decreased pressure in the chest, forces the lymph onward.

Unless you have cardiomyopathy (a failure of the heart muscle to contract), atherosclerosis only forms at the subepicardial level, where there are no muscles to squeeze it along. Matter such as oxidized cholesterol is then deposited on the arterial intima of the subepicardial zone. The longer it stays in the wall of the artery, the greater the reaction. That's why it should hail a cab as soon as possible—and the cab had better be there. If the oxidized cholesterol remains, foam cells must engulf it as a protective shield. But eventually even this won't prevent degeneration of the artery, and atherosclerosis follows.

The lymph flow around the heart is significantly dependent on the pressure variation in the thoracic cavity. Shallow breathing decreases it; exercise and deep breathing can increase it by up to 270 percent. Coronary atherosclerosis is associated with a decreased vital capacity, a lack of exercise, and the other factors noted above. Rarely, it can be caused mainly by heredity, in which case even the most diligent exercise and diet may not prevent it, though they'll go a long way toward retarding it. If a person is born with insufficient lymphatic clearance for the heart, say, then a strict diet, ingestion of antioxidants, and exercise will decrease the consequences of such programming.

HDL has been characterized as "good" lipoprotein and mischaracterized as "good" cholesterol, since it transports cholesterol to the liver for metabolism into acid bile. HDL is elevated in joggers, swimmers, vegetarians, and people lucky enough to be in the "longevity syndrome" group—those who grow old without trouble, no matter what their eating or exercise habits. In children, the ratio of HDL to LDL is 1 to 1. In adults, if the ratio is 1 to 3.5 there is probably little risk of atherosclerosis. But if the ratio is greater than that, and if the HDL isn't maximized—that is, if you don't continue to maintain and even widen the width of the tunnel—then you are at significant risk. And you don't have to be.

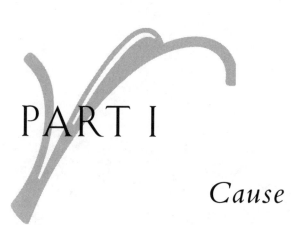

PART I

Cause

1

Cholesterol

Dwight Anderson, seventy-two, a fine osteopathic physician, had a severe, almost fatal heart attack. After he had recovered, he came to see me. I quickly discovered that his cholesterol level was over 270.

I pointed this out to him. "I don't understand why," he said. "I eat only the finest foods at the finest restaurants."

Uh-oh. "No fast foods, then?"

"Greasy killers," he told me self-righteously. "Never touch them."

"These fine restaurants," I said. "What do you tend to eat in them?"

"Lobster's my favorite. The occasional steak or chop."

"*How* occasional?"

"Maybe two, three nights a week."

"Soups?"

"New England clam chowder. Cream of asparagus."

"Cream in your coffee?"

"Mornings and nights. But," he added proudly, "decaf at night. And I know I shouldn't eat ice cream, so I don't."

The conversation is typical. People who eat only "fine" foods, who don't partake of ice cream or french fries, who "wouldn't set foot inside a Burger King or McDonald's," *think* they're eating well but may nevertheless be ingesting cholesterol at a killing rate.

And this is as pernicious as smoking, though far less addictive. Yes, it's fun to eat fatty foods, and I used to think nothing could beat a good steak (now, as I mentioned, it would make me sick). But changing your eating habits can be fun too. This book will show you how.

You are no doubt horrified at tales of chemical companies polluting our rivers. Why are you not horrified when you pollute your internal river, your lymphatics?

GOOD AND BAD CHOLESTEROL

We associate cholesterol primarily with heart disease, and indeed it is one of the major causes—although *only* one—of that potential killer. But other diseases, such as cancer and arthritis, can also be associated with high cholesterol. Patently, it is a dangerous substance and we must be wary of it.

It is also a necessary substance. As we've seen, cholesterol is an essential building block for our cells. When manufactured in the liver (some have called the liver our "metabolic hotel"), it is carried by the bloodstream and deposited wherever cells need regeneration.

Cholesterol, a lipid compound, is also essential for nerve sheaths, for cell membranes, for hormones like cortisone, estrogen, and testosterone. The liver needs it to make bile and the skin to make vitamin D.

However, once cholesterol enters into the wall of the artery, it becomes oxidized and then attracts white cells and tissue growth stimulators into that area of the vessel lining.

Pernicious cholesterol is oxidized cholesterol (technically, having an unpaired electron, it loses an electron). It enters our system via the foods we eat, particularly animal fats and dairy products: steak, chicken, pork; butter, cream, ice cream, milk. (Even though we make 80 percent of our own cholesterol, its production is *stimulated* by the fat we eat.) Inevitably, we will ingest much cholesterol throughout our lives. Some of us can tolerate it far better than others, but all of us should be wary.

Picture yourself driving on a highway. You see a truck in the slow lane delivering cement to an area of the road under repair. Nothing to worry about. You continue driving, your progress unimpeded. If a hundred cement trucks were all unloading their cargo at once, however, the cement would pile up, spill onto the road, and slow your driving—even bring it to a halt.

As with such cement, so with cholesterol. It *is* needed for road repair. Under normal circumstances, the amount that's left over is cleared by the lymphatics. But if an excess of cholesterol appears in the bloodstream—if there's more than the tissue needs or the lymphatics can transport—then the excess spills into the arteries, and if it's not cleared properly, it can cause reactions that will initiate hardening of the arteries.

As we've noted, two types of lipoproteins, the "good" high-density lipoprotein (HDL) and the "bad" low-density lipoprotein (LDL) are important players here. LDL is a large, lightweight, fluffy molecule, much like a microscopic piece of popcorn; HDL is small and smooth like a sunflower seed. Shape is important: HDL is small and pliable enough to pass through the elastic membrane between the inner layer (intima) of the artery wall and into the lymphatic system in the outer layer. LDL, however, cannot pass through the membrane. It is instead broken down into its components in the intima. Its amino acids pass through the membrane and are carried away by the lymphatics, but the fats and cholesterol that remain have to be dealt with. In adults, a ratio of 3.5 to 1 LDL to HDL is considered normal. In sick people the ratio rises from 4.5 to 1 to as high as 8 to 1.

Now, if a large amount of HDL is present in the bloodstream, and thus in the arterial tissue, it will pick up the cholesterol and carry it through to the lymphatics, bringing it into the venous system and then into the liver for breakdown into bile acid, which is excreted into the small intestine. If the bile is passed quickly through the intestines or absorbed by a high-fiber diet, the cholesterol is eliminated. If the bile stays in your system for a long time, however, it is reabsorbed and converted back into cholesterol.

If the cholesterol is *not* picked up by the HDL and carried to the liver, it still has to be taken care of by the body. Unfortunately, when cholesterol reaches the inner wall of the artery, it becomes oxidized—assuming it is not oxidized already—meaning that it has an unpaired electron. That electron needs a mate, which it takes from a normal molecule, thus destroying the healthy components around it. Oxidation renders the cholesterol very dangerous. Platelets and white cells stick to it. This in turn stimulates cell growth, leading to a potentially disastrous thickening of the wall.

The white cells in the wall of the vessel recognize the oxidized cholesterol and ingest it, becoming *foam cells* (white cells that have engulfed cholesterol to prevent it from irritating the tissue). If no method is available for transferring the cholesterol, and the foam cells become so full and aged that they rupture, the cholesterol is scattered into the lining of the artery wall, setting up a tremendous inflammatory reaction. This is the beginning of *arteriosclerotic plaque.*

CHOLESTEROL AND ARTERIOSCLEROSIS

Cholesterol has been implicated as the cause of arteriosclerosis. Indeed, it may be the leading cause. If you have a high level of LDL and not enough HDL to carry it to your liver, an inflammatory reaction is sure to follow, causing arteriosclerosis.

Other causes, however, are also important to consider. I believe that arteriosclerosis is a process of chronic inflammation caused by various agents, working alone or in tandem. You'll see cholesterol involved in all these processes because it is required in the *repair* of the damaged tissues. Thus it has been unfairly blamed as the cause, when in some cases it is an attempt at a cure—it depends on the amount of deposited cholesterol and the amount of HDL available to carry it away, assuming an adequate lymphatic system.

The incidence of arteriosclerosis is high in patients with elevated C-reactive protein levels. C-reactive protein is a marker for inflammation of many kinds and indicates higher risk regardless of cholesterol levels. Patients with arteriosclerosis also have elevated amounts of interleukin-1 (IL-1) and IL-6, proteins found in inflammatory illnesses. Furthermore, some 25 to 30 percent of patients with arteriosclerosis have an elevated homocysteine level, and homocysteine, as we'll see in Chapter 3, is an irritant that can cause an inflammatory process and thereby increase cholesterol deposition at the site of the inflammation.

A correlation is also present between arteriosclerosis and certain infectious processes: dental infections, viral infections, infections with *Chlamydia pneumoniae* and *Helicobacter pylori*, the bacteria that cause stomach ulcers. (Yes, there's a connection between stomach ulcers and heart disease.) Research is still going on in these areas, but I believe that in the near future we'll recognize arteriosclerosis as a multifaceted process, related to an inflammatory response and to a variety of agents, and simply accompanied by a deposition of oxidized cholesterol. Prevention, therefore, should be directed toward removing or avoiding the cause and limiting the inflammation. Oxidative stress, produced by the inflammatory process, can best be diminished by removing the irritants as quickly as possible.

ARTERIOSCLEROSIS AND THE LYMPHATICS

The lymphatic system is closely involved in preventing or reducing this inflammatory process, regardless of its origin. For example, if the primary cause is bacterial or viral in origin, the lymphatics are necessary to recruit appropriate cells and antibodies to destroy the viruses or bacteria. Good lymphatic flow is also essential for the transmission of messenger systems from the affected tissue to the lymph nodes and thymic tissue, which produce bacteria- and virus-resistant cells and substances—a kind of bodily early-warning system. In the case of high cholesterol levels, the lymph is vital in both circulating and increasing the amount of HDL to which the cholesterol can then be exposed. In oxidative stress, it is important for the lymphatics to remove cellular debris from intercellular spaces so that the amount of time it is in contact with the tissue of the arterial wall is limited and the peroxides and free radicals are cleared from the tissue.

I'll be discussing antioxidants in detail later in this book, but it's important now to point out that although nature provides us with antioxidants in every potential situation where oxidative stress can occur—for example, in the lipoprotein that carries cholesterol, a large amount of vitamin E and ubiquinone (also known as coenzyme Q_{10}, or CoQ_{10}) prevent oxidation in the lipids while they are being transported to the tissue—these are sometimes not enough. If we can keep our antioxidant level elevated at the tissue level through diet, exercise, and vitamins, we can reduce the tissue-damaging free radicals that may lead to sometimes fatal inflammation, and the bad effects of oxidized cholesterol can be neutralized.

GOOD CHOLESTEROL, BAD CHOLESTEROL, GOOD FAT, BAD FAT

Although cholesterol can be considered a fat, not all fat contains cholesterol. *Cholesterol is present only in animal tissue,* which is why when you look at a product that proclaims itself "Cholesterol Free," you'll still often find it made up of 45 to 50 percent fat. Vegetable oils, for example, contain no cholesterol; hamburger does. Nevertheless, foods that have no cholesterol (like vegetable oil) can *still* raise your cholesterol count.

The purpose of fat is as a fuel reserve, and when the body sees it, its first reaction is to store it by making new cell membranes to enlarge the fat cells. When fat is eaten, whether or not it contains cholesterol, the body makes extra cholesterol as an essential building block for the manufacture of new cells and maintenance of existing organs. The body manufactures about 80 percent of the cholesterol in our system (we take in only about 300 to 1,000 milligrams a day), and as we've seen, we need it for a variety of purposes.

Current controversy focuses on whether we should have *any* added fat in our diet at all, because all added dietary fats raise our level of cholesterol. Some people feel that even fish oil and vegetable oil can be harmful and recommend we cut them out along with all the animal fats. I think it's true that if we substitute fish oil and vegetable oil for the saturated fats found in foods such as meats, cream, and cheese, we'll still have elevated cholesterol, mainly because the American diet is so fat-heavy anyway (between 35 and 55 percent fat). If we simply substitute vegetable and fish fat for saturated fat, we'll undoubtedly be better off, but we'll still be over-weight and continue to have high cholesterol counts with their attendant problems.

Should we, then, cut out all added fats? I don't think so. I firmly believe that 15 to 20 percent of our diet should be fat, provided it is achieved by a combination of added cold-pressed, extra-virgin olive oil, fish oil, vegetable oil, essential fatty acids, and a small amount of saturated fat, perhaps 1 to 2 percent. Certainly vegetable oils like flaxseed oil, which is high in omega-3 fatty acids, and canola oil can be used in moderation for salads. Vegetable oils should not be used in cooking, however, because they are easily oxidized by heat and can become very dangerous.

Technically, *saturated* fats have hydrogen atoms at each carbon juncture, so that no extra bonds are available between the carbon molecules. This makes them solid at room temperature and more stable when used for cooking. In *polyunsaturated* fats several carbon atoms have an extra electron bond, which makes the fat more liquid at room temperature and allows it to give off more energy (or electrons) in chemical processes, such as heating.

The food industry processes polyunsaturates into saturates by breaking the extra bonds and adding hydrogen—it's how they make margarine, for example. (Such processed polyunsaturated products are called trans-fats.) But these forms of fat are highly toxic. They decrease the production of vitamins, stimulate and oxidize cholesterol, and create oxidative stress. Antioxidants such as vitamins A and E occur naturally in vegetable oils, but when these polyunsaturates are processed, the antioxidants are removed. It's therefore dangerous to ingest large amounts of processed vegetable oil to which no antioxidants have been added; indeed, in those with heart disease and arthritis, such foods may create more damage than saturated fats.

Let me reemphasize the point that *any fats, including manipulated polyunsaturated fats, if taken in the large amounts that the American diet currently contains, will cause problems with cholesterol.* And those problems will lead to chronic diseases such as breast cancer, colon cancer, prostate cancer, and arthritis, to say nothing of arteriosclerosis and heart disease.

ANTIOXIDANTS

We've seen that antioxidants prevent oxidation of cholesterol. They are vital, too, for the production, maintenance, and rejuvenation of our enzyme systems, and they support and assist one another in eliminating the oxidative stress that can lead to harmful free-radical production. Some *water-soluble* antioxidants are vitamin C, albumen, thiol, and bilirubin. *Fat-soluble* antioxidants are vital in the management of cholesterol, as we've seen; examples include vitamin E, vitamin A, and ubiquinone (CoQ_{10}).

Oxidation can be caused by normal cellular respiration, infection, extreme exercise, physical and mental stress, inflammation— and the foods we eat, such as saturated fats and trans-fats. The problem with refined and processed foods is that most of the antioxidants present in them in their natural state are removed during refining or processing. Processed canned food, for example, is always high in sodium because sodium replaces magnesium and potassium—themselves antioxidants—in the processing. Also when we eat refined flour, as in a bagel or white bread, the vitamin E has been removed from the wheat, and no antioxidants are available to counter the stress the flour itself imposes on the body.

FISH AND FLAXSEED,
CHICKEN AND STEAK

Two fatty acids are essential for plasma cell membranes, for certain hormones, and for the regulation of the "messengers" that travel back and forth to activate or deactivate specific cells. These fatty acids are called omega-6 and omega-3. Omega-3 in particular is found in many kinds of fish such as tuna and salmon, in flaxseed oil, and in walnut oil—foods Americans should eat but don't. Instead, we eat steak (thinking that if we cut off the fat, we'll be "watching our cholesterol") and chicken, believing that it is lower in cholesterol than red meat.

In fact, though, both chicken and steak are pernicious when taken in large amounts. (I eat no steak and almost no chicken; Janie eats neither. But I certainly understand the desire for these foods, and an occasional breaking of the rules most likely won't do you much harm.) Removing chicken's skin, with its attendant fat, doesn't really lower the amount of cholesterol you'll ingest, though it will lower the amount of fat. In fact, if you cut the fat off steak, equal portions of this meat and the white meat of chicken will provide about the same amounts of cholesterol.

The optimum level for cholesterol is different for every individual, and it makes no sense to look at these levels in a vacuum. *Remember, it's the* oxidized *cholesterol that's harmful, not cholesterol in general.* Still, as an overall rule, the less cholesterol you eat, the healthier you'll be. "Good" cholesterol, used as unoxidized building blocks of your cell walls, is for the most part manufactured by your own body, and you'll incidentally eat enough in outside foods to supplement it. "Bad" cholesterol must be controlled, and that's up to you.

The regimen I recommend in this book for care of the lymphatic system will keep your cholesterol level down and build up HDL at the expense of LDL. It is by far the best program I can rec-ommend. Still, some of you may want shortcuts—cholesterol-low-ering drugs, cholesterol-free and fat-free foods—and I'll take a moment to discuss these before going on to discuss other dangers to your lymphatic system.

2

"Fat-Free" Foods and Cholesterol-Lowering Drugs

Yesterday I went to my local supermarket to check out fat-free cookies, fat-free cakes, fat-free yogurt, and fat-free ice cream as options for my day's desserts. For breakfast I could have made apple cinnamon muffins from a fat-free mix (0 cholesterol, 130 calories per muffin); for lunch I might have ingested a portion of fat-free raspberry chunk marble ice cream (0 cholesterol, 110 calories per serving) or fat-free frozen vanilla yogurt (0 cholesterol, 70 calories), perhaps garnished with a fat-free devil's food cookie (0 cholesterol, 50 calories); and for dinner consumed a nice slab of angel food cake (0 cholesterol, 140 calories) topped by a scoop of fat-free chocolate ice cream (0 cholesterol, 90 calories) covered with fat-free real chocolate flavor syrup (0 cholesterol, 110 calories).

I settled for melon at breakfast, a mix of blueberries and strawberries for lunch, and no dessert—just green tea—at dinner. I don't trust fat-free foods. Less risky alternatives are out there.

Despite our national obsession with fat-free foods, few consumers take the time to investigate what they are really eating, what—if any—nutritional benefits they are deriving, and whether they might be better off avoiding cookies, cakes, frozen yogurt, and ice cream altogether. Rather, they see "Fat Free" or "Reduced Fat" on the label, eat these products with a feeling of virtue, and proceed with their normal diet, heavy with meat and poultry, thinking that at least they've cut down on fatty foods and given themselves a nutritional boost.

Of course, if they *did* take the time to investigate, they'd soon be mired in confusion. They'd find that some cookies contain no cholesterol, while some double fudge ice cream consists of 13 percent fat and 14 percent cholesterol (to say nothing of 170 calories per serving). They'd find, too, that some (virtually) fat-free foods (shrimp, for example) are high in cholesterol. And some products that label themselves as "Fat Free" (such as cereals and crackers) *shouldn't* have a fat content because they're made from grain. The buyer would be much better off worrying about the amount of sugar they contain, for sugar turns into fat in the body. I suppose the best thing I can say about fat-free foods is that they're better for you than fat-rich foods.

Still, we go on eating foods that are high in fat, such as cheese, meat, and poultry, thinking that by cutting down on other "fatty" foods like cake and ice cream we've done enough in the way of self-care. Then doubt creeps in. Our weight remains constant, or goes up. Unlovable "love handles" appear above our hips. And even worse, our cholesterol level also rises. Four years ago it was at 190. Two years ago it rose to 210, not yet alarming but cause for concern. Now, though, it's at 240 and our internist lectures us. "Too high," she says. "You're putting yourself in harm's way. Better lower your cholesterol, and lower it *now*, or you're in trouble." She writes out a diet high in vegetables and fruits, perhaps prescribes a vitamin and supplement regimen that entails taking more than twenty pills a day, which seems formidable (not to say expensive), and tells us to come back in a year—no more twenty-four months between visits.

But what about the business lunches and dinners, cocktail parties, and afternoon teas featuring Muriel's (all-butter) lemon loaf? What about celebrations, holidays, family get-togethers? Just because our cholesterol is high doesn't mean we should deny our friends and family the food they love—and maybe, to be sociable, partake of it with them just this once.

So our cholesterol levels continue to rise, and now we're in real trouble. We can't seem to change our diets radically enough. On too many occasions, our will power fails. Isn't it time we looked into—indeed, tried—those cholesterol-lowering drugs?

DO DRUGS WORK?

Let's agree on a few basics.

1. It is clear that a high blood cholesterol level is associated with coronary artery disease. It is not the only cause—there are many instances when arteriosclerosis is not associated with cholesterol at all—but it is *a* cause, and it would be foolish not to try to minimize it.
2. If you lower your cholesterol level, you lower your risk of heart attack. Lower your cholesterol by 2 points and your risk of heart attack drops by 1 percent. Lower it by 20 points and your risk drops by 10 percent.
3. It is not, then, a question of *whether* to lower your cholesterol level. It is a question of *how*

Ideally, we can change our diets, increase our exercise, and recenter ourselves to respond healthfully to stress—this book will show you the way. But as we've seen, some people don't have the will, the time, or the inclination, and they look to drugs to do the work for them.

Cholesterol-lowering drugs can stop the progression of plaque formation and, in some cases, actually cause regression of the plaque. This is especially true of "soft plaques," which are vulnerable to cleavage of the planes of cholesterol in the plaque. By reducing the cholesterol in these cleavage planes, the chances of their splitting off and causing obstruction by clot formation is reduced.

But there are side effects—side reactions—particularly if the drugs are used as an excuse for maintaining a high-fat diet throughout the day. Remember: *Cholesterol-lowering drugs should never be employed as a substitute for a low-cholesterol, low-fat diet. They won't work.* Studies have shown that vascular constriction lasts for six to eight hours after eating a high-fat meal. At three meals a day, this means that our vessels would remain in spasm for most of a twenty-four-hour day. Other studies have shown an eight-hour surge of triglycerides and very-low-density lipoproteins (VLDL), both harmful to the artery lining, after a high-fat meal. This isn't prevented by cholesterol-lowering drugs. Indeed, taking them as an antidote to high-fat meals exposes the user to the most serious side effects of these drugs.

Still, I prescribe them from time to time, with substantial benefits to my patients. They're most effective for young people with a high LDL to HDL ratio who have not been able to lower their cholesterol through natural methods. If a six-week "natural" regimen doesn't work, I'll turn to drugs.

KINDS OF CHOLESTEROL-LOWERING DRUGS

Four types of cholesterol-lowering drugs are currently available: niacin, cholestyramine, gemfibrozil, and the "statin" drugs. Each has a different action, different side effects, and a different use in lipid management. Which one is best for you depends on your lipid profile.

NIACIN is a water-soluble B_3 vitamin and is found (in small doses) in most multiple-vitamin capsules. It increases energy and regulates cholesterol and is especially important in good maintenance of the gastrointestinal tract, nervous system, and skin. Mostly it is prescribed for patients with high triglycerides and low HDL.

The daily requirement of niacin for everyone is about 20 milligrams. One-half comes directly from niacin in the diet; the body manufactures the rest from the amino acid tryptophan, found in meat, fish, eggs, and some vegetables.

It is only when taken in higher doses, from 100 to 2,000 milligrams, that niacin acts as a cholesterol-lowering drug. It is effective in raising HDL and lowering LDL and VLDL and is especially valuable in treating high triglycerides. It also acts as an artery and blood vessel relaxer. But beware: these benefits are derived from niacin (nicotinic acid), not niacinamide, another form of B_3.

The primary side effects of using niacin to lower cholesterol include skin flushing, tingling, and, especially serious, liver dysfunction. Therefore you should have your liver function checked before you start on this therapy, particularly if you plan to be on it for a long time. (Treatments can last from six months to a year, depending on the case.) Under no circumstances should you use time-released niacin, the form with which liver problems are most

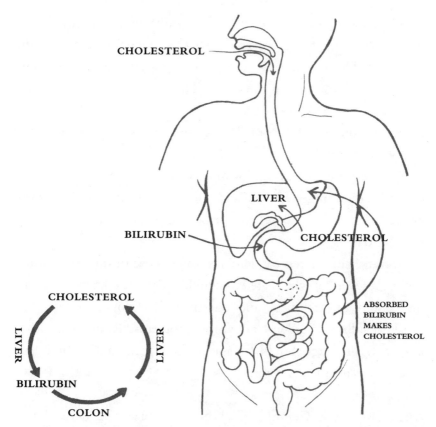

CHOLESTEROL

LIVER

BILIRUBIN

CHOLESTEROL

ABSORBED
BILIRUBIN
MAKES
CHOLESTEROL

CHOLESTEROL

LIVER

LIVER

BILIRUBIN

COLON

Diagram of cholesterol cycle in the human body

frequently encountered. Skin flushing can be managed by slowly building up the level of niacin, taking an aspirin half an hour before use, or taking niacin with meals. A "flush-free" form of niacin called inositol hexaniacinate is available but is not always effective.

Niacin can also precipitate gout, increase blood sugar in diabetics, and cause hypotension in patients being treated with antihypertensive medications.

CHOLESTYRAMINE, also known as Questran or Cholybar, acts by binding the bile in the small bowel and extracting it in the stool.

It's like an artificial high-fiber diet. A significant amount of cholesterol is converted to bile salts by the liver and then secreted into the bile duct. The cholesterol next passes through the bowel, where finally it is reabsorbed in the colon. This internal shunt of cholesterol is broken by cholestyramine so that the cholesterol, instead of reentering the blood to contribute to the cholesterol level, is passed out of the body.

Cholestyramine can significantly lower the cholesterol level. It can also bind ingested fats and vitamins, so it must be given between meals to allow for prior absorption of macro- and micronutrients.

Adverse side effects can also accompany use of this medication, the most severe of which are fat-soluble vitamin deficiencies, bloating, distension, gassiness, and constipation. Long-term use may cause bleeding disorders and vision problems. Remember, it's a *drug,* and all drugs should be approached with caution and only under a doctor's supervision.

GEMFIBROZIL Gemfibrozil (Lopid), a fibric acid derivative, is particularly useful because it lowers triglycerides without the flushing caused by niacin. It, too, is a high-fiber substitute. It has been shown to elevate HDL without affecting LDL and has thus been found effective in patients with low HDL levels. It can, however, cause achy and inflamed muscles; it may be carcinogenic; and, in combination with the "statin" drugs, it can be followed (on rare occasions) by complete muscle breakdown.

"STATIN" DRUGS The "statin" drugs—e.g., simvastatin (Zocor), pravastatin (Pravachol), lovastatin (Mevacor), atorvastatin (Lipitor)—are perhaps the most effective— and most dangerous— of the cholesterol-lowering drugs. They block one of the enzymes that creates cholesterol.

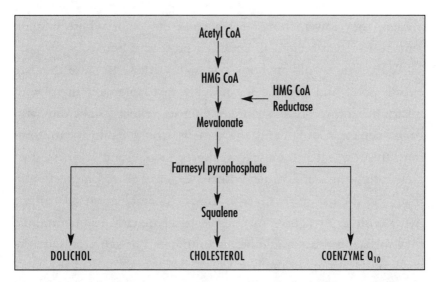

Schematic representation of the biosynthetic pathway leading to cholesterol, dolichol, and coenzyme Q_{10}

The problem is that they also block the production of other essential compounds, such as CoQ_{10}, which is both a powerful antioxidant and a bioenergy producer necessary for the mitochondria of the cells to produce fuel important to bodily functions.

Loss of CoQ_{10} can affect the immune system, causing heart failure, among other disorders. Hypersensitivity reactions may also occur, leading to pneumonitis, rashes, cardiomyopathy, fatigability, joint pain, psoriasis, shortness of breath, and swelling of feet and hands. Such symptoms have been seen in some 7.7 percent of the patients who take statin drugs. Liver failure, gallbladder disease, and lupuslike symptoms have also been reported, along with common complaints of discomfort, gassiness, bloating, and cramps. Early studies of the statin drugs reported a higher incidence of cancer (researchers at the University of San Francisco found that the statins are carcinogenic in animals), suicide, and mental instability. Some doctors have associated the statin drugs with Alzheimer's disease because they lower cholesterol beyond the point where enough remains to repair brain cells and their protective linings.

Why, then, would anybody take statin drugs? Because they are effective, yes, and because it's possible to supplement them with micronutrients to prevent some of their side effects. Since the statin drugs deplete CoQ_{10}, and the patient would exhibit symptoms from this loss, such as muscle weakness, fatigue, and soreness, supplementing the statin drugs with CoQ_{10} has proved protective in many cases. If patients who have tried this combination still suffer a hypersensitivity reaction, manifested by hives, rash, or pneumonia, then the statin drug should be discontinued. The symptoms are the result of the drug, not the CoQ_{10}.

In all cases, be careful. The statin drugs have been loudly and widely advertised—it's hard to spend an evening in front of the tube without seeing an ad for, say, Lipitor—but the possible harmful side effects (mentioned in a low voice or in small print) are downplayed, when to my mind they should be stressed.

Still, Dr. Stephen Sinatra, a cardiologist and bioenergetic analyst who runs the New England Heart Center, is a firm believer in the use of 10 to 20 milligrams of pravastatin a day, at least for some women with a history of heart disease and high cholesterol levels. "I am convinced," he writes, "of its ability to prevent heart attack, bypass surgery, angioplasty, stroke and even death, particularly in women who fit this profile; that is, women who are at high risk and cannot reduce their cholesterol by natural means." The drug has worked with men, too, he continues, but the research demonstrates that women do significantly better on this therapy. (He warns, though, that 12 of 576 women taking pravastatin in a recent trial developed breast cancer, and while it is not clear that pravastatin was the culprit, he suggests that women with a family history of cancer first discuss the use of pravastatin with their doctors.) On occasion when he does have to prescribe a statin drug, he strongly recommends at least 100 to 200 milligrams of CoQ_{10} a day.

CASE HISTORIES

A NATIONALLY KNOWN dog trainer and world traveler, who just happened to be eighty-one, went for her first medical checkup in a decade "because it was time." She was in perfect health except for her total cholesterol, which was 227. Her doctor immediately put her on Zocor. In the next four to five weeks she developed hair loss, loss of balance, and overall weakness, and so she called me. I recommended she stop Zocor, and almost immediately all her symptoms disappeared. She has been on my cholesterol-reducing program since then, and now her cholesterol is below 200. None of her symptoms has returned.

A SIXTY-NINE-YEAR-OLD WOMAN with a history of hypertension and type II diabetes mellitus came to a clinic for evaluation of a recent cough. She had been taking 20 to 40 milligrams of pravastatin daily for six years, along with a battery of medications to treat her other ailments. Despite a negative radiograph and sinus computed tomography (CT) scan, a potent nasal spray and the drug loratidine (Claritin) were then added to her medicines. However, since she continued to cough, she was next started on prednisone. Her symptoms worsened further; the prednisone was stopped. An open-lung biopsy revealed hypersensitivity pneumonitis. The pravastatin was finally stopped. Her cough disappeared in two weeks. A follow-up high-resolution scan seven weeks after the first one showed no sign of pneumonitis.

A SIXTY-SIX-YEAR-OLD MAN was found to need a six-vessel bypass as treatment for severe coronary heart disease. Afterward a daily dose of 20 milligrams of lovastatin was given for moderately severe lipid abnormalities. Four years later the patient complained of fatigue, somnolence, and joint pain. His shortness of breath continued despite the use of dexamethasone and bronchodilators. Only after the lovastatin was discontinued did his symptoms disappear.

A SEVENTY-SIX-YEAR-OLD WOMAN had an aortic valve replacement along with coronary artery bypass surgery. Immediately afterward she was started on 20 milligrams of lovastatin daily, and one year later she began to complain of muscle aches. Two years after that she developed joint pain, followed by psoriasis. Despite nonsteroidal anti–inflammatory drug therapy, steroids, and methotrexate, she worsened and began to experience shortness of breath. Inhaled steroids and bronchodilators were prescribed. She then complained of back pain and depression. Finally lovastatin was discontinued, and over a two-month period, all her symptoms gradually improved.

A FIFTY-THREE-YEAR-OLD MAN with a history of coronary angioplasty developed angioedema (swelling) of the eyelids within six months of beginning to take pravastatin (40 milligrams daily). He took diphenhydramine for relief, along with isosorbide mononitrate, diltiazem, aspirin, alprazolam, and multivitamins. His serum complement, blood count, sedimentation rate, and antinuclear antibodies tests (for allergies) were normal. But only after he stopped taking the pravastatin did his symptoms gradually resolve.

A FRIEND and colleague of mine, T.R., had a cholesterol level of 290 with high LDL and low HDL, despite the fact that he ate a healthy diet, exercised regularly, was far from overweight, and didn't smoke. (Maybe he led too stressful a life or had a genetic predisposition to high cholesterol.) I put him on a statin drug regimen, and his cholesterol dropped to 150, where it is now.

WHAT DOES IT ALL MEAN?

Adverse reactions occur in only a small percentage (7.7 percent) of cholesterol-lowering drug users, generally require exposure to the same or chemically related drugs, develop rapidly after reexposure, and produce clinical syndromes similar to those commonly associated with immunologic reactions. In all of these instances, such symptoms improve markedly once the drug is stopped.

You'll note that these case studies involve older patients, but the elderly are not the only people at risk. One of my patients, a thirty-seven-year-old advertising executive, took drugs to lower a cholesterol level of 240 and almost immediately suffered aches and pains all over his body.

In my opinion, cholesterol-lowering drugs should be used only when all natural methods fail. I *urge* my patients to avoid the drugs whenever possible and to follow my program instead. Diet, exercise, stress reduction, and vitamins are not "alternative" medicines or a substitute for medicine. They *are* medicines and are often more powerful, less potentially injurious, and far more benign than the more conventional pharmacological solutions.

Besides, as I have argued, factors exclusive of cholesterol may well be the underlying cause of arteriosclerosis, and the panoply of drugs the cholesterol "industry" has engendered does not address these. Perhaps the most prevalent current example of such a contributor is homocysteine, as we shall see next.

3

Homocysteine

D
r. Carl Steel came to see me for a consultation. An internist and hematologist by training, at age fifty-five he was plagued by angina. Several angioplasties had done nothing to relieve the pain, nor had enrollment in a world-famous West Coast program of vegetarian diet, exercise, and stress management. One last angioplasty had failed, and now he was desperate.

I suggested he might have an elevated homocysteine level.

"What's that?" he asked, surprised.

I explained that homocysteine was an amino acid that caused plaque formation, clotting, platelet stickiness, and spasm of the endothelium of the vessel walls. "Let's take a blood level for homocysteine," I told him, "and see what we find."

As I expected, Dr. Steel's homocysteine level was high. I prescribed the vitamins and minerals you will find recommended in this book. Within weeks his pain had disappeared. As of now, four years later, it has not reappeared.

AMINO ACIDS

Amino acids are the building blocks of the proteins in our bodies. Protein, in turn, is necessary for the strength of muscle tissue, including the heart muscle. Yet the body itself cannot manufacture the essential amino acids; they must be taken in through the food we eat. One such amino acid, methionine, is found in many meat and dairy products; it is in the metabolism of methionine that homocysteine is manufactured.

Homocysteine is an amino acid produced by the body in minute amounts. It is normally then converted into compounds the body needs (such as cysteine and adenosine triphosphate), changed back to methionine, or—through transfer of a sulfur molecule—transformed into glutathione, a nontoxic amino acid. If such conversion does not occur, however, intact homocysteine causes an increase in platelet stickiness and clumping and promotes the oxidation of lipids like LDL, thereby causing damage to the inner lining of arterial walls. Eventually arteriosclerosis, tissue degeneration, and blood clots may follow.

Vitamin B_6, folic acid, and vitamin B_{12} are necessary for this amino acid transformation process. Unfortunately, about 12 percent of the U.S. population has an inborn metabolic flaw that prevents the full metabolization of homocysteine, and the elderly are particularly deficient in these B vitamins. It is therefore easy for many people's homocysteine levels to build up dangerously. Indeed, in June 1997 the *New England Journal of Medicine* acknowledged that "an increased homocysteine level confirms an independent risk of vascular disease similar to that of smoking. It powerfully increases the risk associated with smoking and hypertension." Therefore we test for and treat elevated homocysteine levels.

HOMOCYSTEINE AND ARTERIOSCLEROSIS

One reason homocysteine is so dangerous is that it is a silent enemy; it may produce no symptoms for a long time. The public is generally unaware of it, partly because it has received little publicity through advertising by the drug companies—in contrast to the fanfare surrounding cholesterol. (I imagine that if a drug existed, costing $1,500 a year, that reduced homocysteine levels, we'd hear about it—loudly.) Also the tests for homocysteine level are expensive—about $100 per test—and are not yet routinely done at most hospitals. These assessments must be sent to a commercial laboratory, and it often takes weeks for the results to come back. Indeed, only recently has the medical profession in general become cognizant of homocysteine's importance, and the story explaining that is a complex and unpleasant one.

In 1969 a Harvard pathologist, Dr. Kilmer McCulley, observed that homocysteinemia, regardless of its origin, was associated with early arteriosclerosis. Indeed, he postulated that virtually *all* arteriosclerosis is caused by a metabolic excess of homocysteine. Cholesterol, McCulley argued, is simply a symptom of arteriosclerosis, not a cause, and in fact all the research done on cholesterol has never actually proven a causal relationship between high cholesterol levels and arteriosclerosis, only a strong correlation. McCulley's interest was piqued by studying the autopsy reports on two children suffering from homocysteinuria, a rare genetic disorder in which the liver cannot break down homocysteine into harmless components. Both children died of heart attacks due to arteriosclerosis, and they should have been sixty or seventy years older to have perished in such a fashion.

In further studies, McCulley discovered that increased homocysteine directly inflamed the inner linings of arterial walls, leading to the buildup of atherosclerotic plaque. Indeed, after injecting rabbits with homocysteine, he found that such plaques developed in their coronary arteries within weeks.

Since methionine is found in meat and animal products, McCulley proposed that eating too much of these foods might cause damage not because of the amount of cholesterol they contained (the argument many doctors and dietitians have used in urging a reduction in meat and dairy consumption) but because of their high levels of methionine. The American diet of meat, dairy products, and canned, boxed, processed, or preserved foods was dangerous, he said, because it was depriving us, among other things, of the B vitamins essential for combating the buildup of homocysteine.

The medical professionals—to say nothing of the drug industry—came down hard on him, particularly those who were already committed to the cholesterol theory of arteriosclerosis. They approved of his dietary recommendations but not his reasoning. Even when, in 1976, Australian researchers published a study showing a definite connection between high homocysteine levels and heart disease in humans, and McCulley's studies with rabbits had been confirmed in baboons (which are more similar to humans), the National Institutes of Health did not renew the grants for his research. He was forced to cut down his staff and eventually to leave Massachusetts General Hospital, where he had done his research, thus ending his tenure at Harvard as well.

The full story of the medical blackballing of Dr. McCulley, which continued for nearly thirty years, has no place in this book, but I still get angry when I think of it. I myself experienced such treatment when my colleagues at first refused to refer patients to me once I began advocating a fruit, vegetable, and vitamin regimen for the prevention and treatment of coronary heart disease. Still, the treatment McCulley received at the hands of the medical establishment was a thousand times worse. Eventually, thanks to the intervention of a leading Boston lawyer, the vilification lessened and he was able to work at the Veterans Administration Hospital in Providence, Rhode Island. At present he is exploring the possible relationship between homocysteine and other severe illnesses such as stroke and cancer.

By now his theory that homocysteine can cause hardening of the arteries has been accepted. The question is no longer *whether* but to *what degree* homocysteine plays a role in arteriosclerosis. Which is the most important real offender, the argument rages, homocysteine or cholesterol?

THE CHANGING CULPRIT

Fifty years ago, research was begun on residents of Framingham, Massachusetts, to see if any common factors were associated with increased rates of heart attacks. As the study progressed, it was clear that those with elevated cholesterol levels and high blood pressure, or hypertension, were most at risk. If they were also smokers, their danger was even greater. The conclusion was clear: the way to prevent heart attacks was to bring down cholesterol and blood pressure, control weight, and encourage people to give up cigarettes. This became—and still is—the conventional medical wisdom.

Because of the Framingham study's findings, the massive Multiple Risk Factor Intervention Trial was instituted at medical centers throughout the country, designed to eliminate these causes. Yet after seven years, although the "villains" were in fact dramatically reduced, *no concomitant drop in the rates of heart attack followed*.

Indeed, when it comes to cholesterol, for example, a larger and larger body of research suggests that there is no proof that lowering cholesterol can save lives, particularly in people over the age of sixty-five. Too low cholesterol levels in the aged can even lead to behavioral changes, including depression and suicide. Furthermore, cholesterol-lowering drugs may be harmful if used as an essential and not in the context of a low-fat diet. In children, cholesterol is an essential component of several important hormones and other steroids. Therefore a child should only take cholesterol-lowering drugs in a severely unmanageable case. Cutting out milk and ice cream, say, for lowering cholesterol in growing children may be counterproductive.

When data from the Framingham study were looked at more deeply, a clear correlation did appear between homocysteine levels and the amount of arteriosclerosis in the arteries. In a different ongoing study, it was discovered that higher homocysteine levels were a better predictor of heart attacks than elevated cholesterol. *It is now believed that homocysteine levels may be some 40 percent more accurate than cholesterol levels for predicting heart disease.* Indeed, homocysteine is associated with cardiovascular disease in up to 30 percent of patients. Dr. McCulley, it would seem, was not the crackpot he was made out to be.

My own view is that *both* oxidized cholesterol and homocysteine—among many other elements—are causative factors in arteriosclerosis. One can easily see how the two can be confounded, since most of the food high in cholesterol is also high in methionine. The vitamin B deficiency attendant on high homocysteine levels can also affect cholesterol levels because B vitamins are necessary in the manufacture of antioxidants, essential fatty acids, and other components of the body that can detoxify cholesterol.

The problem with either theory is that it is not universally applicable. As noted, no studies have proved conclusively that lowering dietary cholesterol cuts down the risk of heart disease, let alone eliminates it; and I personally have seen many patients with significant coronary or vascular disease who have normal homocysteine levels.

TESTING FOR HOMOCYSTEINE

Two screening methods are currently available to determine whether you have too much homocysteine in your blood. The fasting blood homocysteine level is a good screening test, but perhaps a superior method is a methionine tolerance test, in which you are given a methionine load and your blood levels are measured afterward; this is performed much like a glucose tolerance test. Both homocysteine tests are expensive and therefore probably should not be used as is in screening the general public.

I don't currently order fasting blood homocysteine on patients except under the following conditions:

- A family history of homocysteinemia is present. (For some reason, this occurs most frequently in patients with an Irish background).
- Hardening of the arteries has appeared in multiple places, such as the carotids, heart, and/or legs.
- Onset hardening of the arteries has developed in patients below age fifty.
- A previous bypass procedure has led to an early graft closure.
- Arteriosclerosis is present even in the face of low cholesterol and/or high HDL.

LOWERING HOMOCYSTEINE

I approach the treatment of homocysteine with a three-pronged attack. The first step involves reduction of methionine in the diet and the addition of vitamins B_6, B_{12}, and folic acid to minimize the amount of homocysteine that's converted from the methionine. The second is to supply antioxidants, such as vitamins C and E, to prevent the oxidative stress caused by homocysteine in the vessel wall. The third is to increase lymphatic flow, so that the products of methionine and the reactive biochemicals formed by the interaction of homocysteine with the body tissues are rapidly cleared by way of the lymphatics, then broken down by the liver.

Step 1: Reducing Methionine

We can't completely eliminate methionine from our diet, nor would we want to. But we *can* cut down on dairy products and red meat. A 12-ounce steak feeds a family of four in China; here it feeds one. Most third world countries, where arteriosclerosis is not a large-scale problem, eat primarily vegetables and fish. Further:

- Substitute soy or rice milk for cow's milk. A strong correlation exists between casein (the protein in milk), lactose (the sugar in milk), and heart disease. Furthermore, when milk is homogenized, xanthine oxidase is absorbed into the bloodstream along with the fat. This is a particularly harmful enzyme that causes tissue damage and the release of free radicals.
- Discontinue caffeine and coffee drinking.
- Increase the amount of fresh fruits and vegetables in your

diet. They supply the necessary vitamins, B_6, B_{12}, and folic acid, to contend with the homocysteine.

- Minimize processed foods. They just add calories without any of the necessary micronutrients.
- Supplement with B_6, B_{12}, and folic acid to convert the homocysteine in the system back to methionine or transform it into innocuous amino acids such as glutathione. (I will discuss the amount I recommend in the following section.)

Step 2: Preventing Oxidative Stress

The second part of our plan is to minimize the noxious effects of homocysteine at the tissue level by reducing oxidative stress and its subsequent inflammatory process.

- Add the antioxidant vitamins A, C, and E to your diet, both by supplementation and through a diet of unprocessed vegetables and fruits.
- Limit the inflammatory reaction by the ingestion of omega-3 fatty acids. Eat cold-water fatty fish such as salmon, tuna, and halibut, or supplement with 3 grams of omega-3 fatty acids per day; vegetarians may substitute flaxseed oil.
- Take magnesium, zinc, calcium, and selenium, which serve as catalysts in the body's enzyme processes, helping it manufacture its essential enzymes and antioxidants.

Step 3: Increasing Lymphatic Drainage

As I have said, this is a vital process that clears the initiating toxins and the intermediate oxidative radicals from the tissue, thus minimizing their damage. Its methods include deep breathing, stress modification, exercise—indeed, the entire program laid out in this book.

MORE ON SUPPLEMENTS

Overall, I think it unwise to believe that a diet without supplements can provide all the B vitamins we need to counter the effects of methionine. Even taking B vitamin supplements to bring us up to the recommended daily allowance (RDA) may not be enough. I've seen cases where only heightened dosages of B_6 and folic acid have led to a drop in the homocysteine level. These same patients, on a standard vitamin B regimen, have tested for homocysteine levels of 15 μmol/dl or greater, whereas 8 μmol/dl is optimum. The figures on pages 60 and 61 show how vitamins B_6, B_{12}, and folic acid can convert homocysteine into its healthful by-products.

Another such transforming agent is trimethylglycine (TMG), which must be taken in tablet form. TMG helps methylate the homocysteine back to methionine, then to be metabolized. I think TMG is important, especially in older people, because their decreased gastric acidity cannot absorb vitamin B_{12} from the diet. Betaine, a substance found in sugar beets, also helps prevent aging, atherosclerosis, and cancer by protecting DNA from damage. Since TMG and betaine affect different pathways, their combination produces a synergistic effect. Some people need more of one than the other because of faulty diet and genetic enzymatic defects. And remember: homocysteine levels rise with age and are affected by alcohol, synthetic estrogen, chemotherapy, and other drugs that interfere with vitamin B.

The daily requirement for prevention of elevated homocysteine levels in patients without homocysteinemia is 3 milligrams of B_6 and 400 micrograms of folic acid daily. I also add 1,000 milligrams

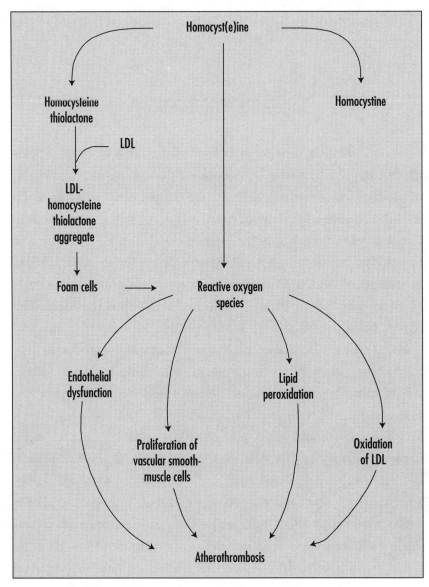

Source: *New England Journal of Medicine*

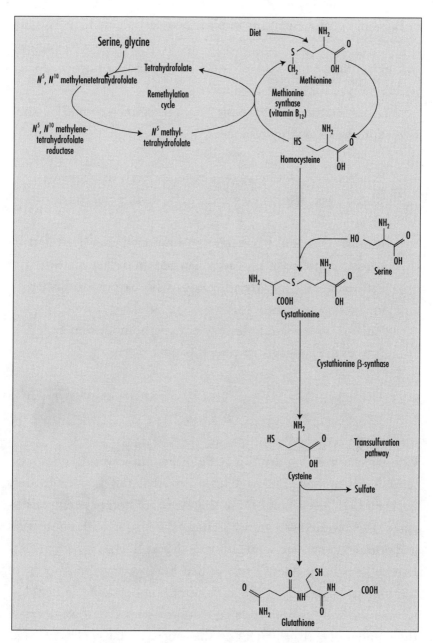

Source: *New England Journal of Medicine*

of B_{12} sublingually, especially in older people, because their low gastric acidity prevents absorption of B_{12} from their food. I increase this by tenfold when patients do not respond to normal dosage with a drop in homocysteine levels.

Further increases of this basic vitamin regimen should be considered in the following instances:

- Patients with elevated homocysteine levels to begin with whose levels remain elevated or rise despite the usual formula
- Patients who still have elevated homocysteine levels and coronary disease in the face of an optimum diet
- Patients at risk for arteriosclerosis who have poor dietary intake
- Patients with a family history of hyperhomocysteinemia
- Any of the above in an elderly patient

DRUGS

Cholesterol-lowering drugs may be of help in lowering homocysteine levels as well. Dr. McCulley says that this is because they decrease LDL levels, and LDL is the carrier of homocysteine. I disagree. LDL is merely a transportation system for both cholesterol and homocysteine, and while it's true that LDL goes up when cholesterol goes up, it doesn't follow that by lowering the amount of transportation you lower the amount of homocysteine and cholesterol in the body as well. It's analogous to saying that if we decrease the number of garbage trucks on the streets, we'll have less garbage, and this obviously isn't the case. We'll have less garbage removed from the house, but it will build up in the house all the same. Less homocysteine will be carried by the LDL whenever the LDL is reduced, but it remains a danger to the system nevertheless.

Are there specific homocysteine-lowering drugs? Not yet, although I can envision a time when drug and fruit and vegetable companies will bombard our shelves with "methionine blockers" and "methionine-free" meats and ice cream. But, as we've seen, methionine, like cholesterol, is necessary for essential bodily processes, and we must be cautious before we rush to lower or eliminate it.

A RANGE OF CULPRITS

In truth, a range of causes may contribute to arteriosclerosis, and unless further research leads to increased specificity, the cholesterol/homocysteine debate is largely academic. Both should be monitored throughout your lifetime.

It is helpful, I think, to look at arteriosclerosis much like a rash on the skin. Rashes can be caused by many agents: bacteria, viruses, allergens, poisons, even psychological problems and stress. In other words, a rash is a rash, but the irritating agent may be different in each case. Similarly, arteriosclerosis can be caused by oxidized cholesterol, homocysteine, cellular breakdown products, trauma, bacteria, viruses, and probably other agents to date unknown. Also, stress and psychological problems may add to the difficulty. I'll discuss all of these more fully in the next chapter.

IN BRIEF

The best approach to reducing the danger of arteriosclerosis from homocysteinemia is to:

1. Minimize the ingestion and production of homocysteine.
2. Maximize the antioxidants and anti-inflammatory defenses in your body.
3. Optimize the lymphatic flow from your arterial tissues to clear them of any irritating agents and intermediate metabolites that might go on to produce arteriosclerosis.

The program in this book, besides diminishing your risk for arteriosclerosis, also reduces your chances of phlebitis, inflammation of the veins, and any clotting problem such as stroke or pulmonary embolus.

4

Toxic Substances

I read of a woman recently diagnosed with breast cancer. When her tumor was biopsied, her doctors found something extraordinary: a large deposit of DDT. *Yet DDT has been outlawed for over twenty years. It had remained in her tissue for all that time, resulting in the malignancy.*

Anything that causes a harmful reaction when introduced into the body can be termed a *toxic substance*. It may be a living organism—a bacterium or a virus, say—or an organic (DDT, PVC, dioxin) or inorganic material (asbestos or a variety of poisons). It can even be a by-product of the body's own metabolic processes: homocysteine, as we've seen, can be extremely toxic, as can cholesterol and lactic acid.

For the purposes of this book, when I discuss toxic substances I am talking about those that are ingested or inhaled and, through a series of events, cause a chronic degenerative disease such as arteriosclerosis, cancer, or arthritis. These toxic agents can affect the lymphatic system as well as many other bodily functions. Such irritants do not automatically disappear in the lymphatics. However, the more cleanly flowing your lymphatic system the more likely it is that they will be carried to the liver where they can be metabolized or excreted through the urine.

For example, women who wear bras don't have normal movement in their breast tissue. As a result, their lymphatics slow, and toxins stay in the tissue. This can cause changes in the DNA, which may cause cancer. A Swedish study showed not only a strong correlation between cancer of the breast and the wearing of brassieres but also a twenty-nine-fold decrease in the breast cancer rates when women went without this undergarment. Therefore it's a good policy for women to go without a brassiere for at least several hours a day. A series of exercises, arm stretching, and massaging the quadrants of the breast can also benefit lymphatic flow in the breast. (It is imprudent, however, to massage breasts in the presence or suspected presence of cancer because it may increase the spread of the cancer cells.)

In medicine, it sometimes seems, every "healthy" regimen has its danger. Toxins can accrue from so normal an exercise as running. In extremely energetic runners, a buildup of lactic acid and oxidative products occurs. Lactic acid will eventually be converted into carbon dioxide and water and subsequently be excreted, but while it remains in the tissue it's a strong irritant. This accumulation explains why we get muscle cramps after strenuous activity. Massage is the best antidote, for it helps move the lactic acid from the tissue into the lymphatic flow.

THE EFFECTS OF TOXIC SUBSTANCES

Toxic substances can harm the body in three ways:

1. When ingested, they can directly damage the cells.
2. When a toxic buildup develops within the body, the body's metabolism can produce a harmful reaction as it attempts to clear the substance.
3. The substance can react within the cells, and the cells themselves produce a harmful by-product as a result of and in reaction to contact with the toxins.

The fact that toxic substances can be ingested or produced within the body whenever the metabolism is in a deficiency state is a vital concept to underscore when we look for the cures to chronic degenerative diseases. For these diseases—including arteriosclerosis—can develop only if an initiating factor intrudes from outside the body or a toxic substance is produced from within.

TOXIC SUBSTANCES AND ARTERIOSCLEROSIS

Many toxic materials can initiate the inflammatory process we know as arteriosclerosis. Most commonly we think of cholesterol as the chief offending agent, but many others may create disease. When the body is threatened with a toxic substance, it will defend itself through the manufacture of antioxidants and vitamins at the tissue level that can neutralize or detoxify the substance. Still, the substance must be carried away, and that is the job of the lymphatics. If the toxic load is too great, the antioxidants at the tissue level insufficient, or the lymphatic clearance inadequate, this is a setup not only for arteriosclerosis but for many other degenerative diseases.

Toxic substances can either be directly destroyed by medicines, as in the case of bacteria or viruses, or detoxified, usually by adding a methyl (CH_3) group, 4-carbon methyl group, or a sulfur atom, so that the perpetrator is not as deadly to cells and can be more easily excreted through the kidney or the liver.

These helpful biochemical reactions take place at the cell level and in the interstitial spaces. Any by-products of these events, along with any remaining toxins, are then passed from the interstitial spaces into the lymphatic collecting ducts and on into the lymphatics. How long these toxic substances and their by-products stay in the interstitial spaces determines the amount of inflammatory reaction or mutation of the genetic material in the cell that will take place. Thus it's best to get rid of them quickly—a prime reason why a smoothly functioning, cleanly flowing lymph system is so vital to your good health.

MAN-MADE TOXINS

Toxins can have many effects, depending on their local cell reaction and method of removal from the body. But one constant remains: all toxins are cleared from the tissue to the kidney or liver through the lymphatics. The danger here is that some toxins can destroy the liver or kidneys—mercury, for example, or lead, man-made toxins as lethal as the most virulent virus. The particular problem with heavy metals is that there is no way to excrete them; they must be absorbed and accumulated within the body. Once they end up in the nervous system, they can cause severe nervous disorders.

Mercury is concentrated in fish, especially older, larger fish, which have ingested it from the spillage of chemical plants into our rivers and oceans. For this reason, I believe that it's wise to avoid eating swordfish steaks, large tuna, and shark meat; these fish may have lived as long as twenty years. Since no animal or fish can excrete the mercury it takes in, any other animal that chows down on these creatures will also be ingesting their mercury intake, and so on up the line. My advice therefore is to eat as little meat as possible, and when choosing fish, to stick with young salmon or halibut.

Lead is a toxic substance, once found in paint, and gasoline, that can cause neurological problems. Lead or mercury poisoning is often treated by a process called *chelation*, in which the chelating agent, called EDTA, can, like a crab, grab and hold heavy metal in place in the body and allow it to be processed by the kidney and ultimately excreted. Short of this—and no absolute proof exists that chelating works, even though it has been used for almost fifty years—no real method is yet available for excreting metals like lead, mercury, and aluminum from the body.

Chlorine is a highly toxic element that causes oxidative stress when introduced into the body. Children are particularly sensitive to it, and those parents who don't let their children swim in chlorinated pools are probably being prudent.

Inhaled toxins such as smoke (cigarette or industrial), smog, and petrochemicals cause tremendous oxidative stress at the local tissue level within the lungs. This then creates an inflammatory reaction leading to breakdown of the whole adjacent area. The result? Obstructive pulmonary disease, emphysema, even—if a genetic change develops in the cells—lung cancer.

The insecticides of the 1940s, 1950s, and 1960s were particularly harmful to tissues, and many people are still feeling the aftereffects of their use. I started the chapter with an example of a woman whose cancer was the direct result of one of these chemicals, DDT, and the wonder is now why scientists did not recognize that a chemical compound used to kill bugs would not have deleterious effects on people, too.

It fascinates me that trace elements of these compounds can be found in biopsy tissue of patients twenty to thirty years after the chemical has been taken off the market. The reason, I have concluded, is that these petrochemicals are fat-soluble and are carried to the fatty tissue for storage. If your lymphatic flow is not optimal, they stay in the fat tissue, cause genetic changes to the DNA of the cells, and lead to cancer many years later.

THE IMMUNE SYSTEM

To understand the effects of toxins, we have to look at how the immune system works. Immunity can be either specific or nonspecific. Nonspecific immunity is our body's reaction to any outside substance not derived from itself. The body can recognize a foreign protein or organism and has the innate ability to attack and destroy that material. Specific immunity is then evoked from our body's memory of having been introduced to the outside toxic substance in the past. The body stores in its cells and fluids ways to react against that specific outside invader, and when it encounters the substance again, it attacks.

These two types of specific immunity are called *cell-mediated* and *humoral* immunity. Cell-mediated immunity is the process by which the cells directly engage with the outside substances, attacking and destroying them. In humoral immunity, our body recognizes the foreign substance and then creates antibodies to circulate in the body fluids, which will attach to any invading substance and destroy it. This ability is based on the recognition by the body of the foreign substance—its "memory."

Cells that create antibodies are called plasma cells. They identify a foreign substance and then manufacture a Y-shaped protein that will lock onto the foreign invader and destroy it. These antibodies float freely in the blood and lymphatic systems and are also attached to the membrane of the plasma cell, so that when they come into contact with the toxic substance they can lock the plasma cell onto it. Plasma cells live in the lymphatic system and lymph nodes. They are formed from B cells, white cells that live in the spleen, bone marrow, liver, and thymus.

The Antibodies

Five main classes of antibodies can be distinguished, with a different purpose for each class.

1. Immunoglobulin G (IgG) antibodies pursue antigens and are the most common type found in the body. They are produced late in the immune response, so that when they're seen, it's a sign of an ongoing or established infection.

2. Immunoglobulin M (IgM) antibodies signal recent infection. They are initially mobilized when a pathogen invades the body and peaks in several weeks.

3. Immunoglobulin E (IgE) antibodies come into play in allergic reactions such as asthma, eczema, and hay fever.

4. Immunoglobulin A (IgA) antibodies are found in saliva, tears, and the mucous membranes of the gastrointestinal tract. They are a defense against proteins and bacteria invading the mucosa or the bowels. These antibodies disappear whenever the secretions of the gut are decreased. Proper diet or, in some severe cases, medicine will help eliminate any underlying problem responsible for their excess production.

5. The fifth antibody, known as immunoglobin D (IgD), is a little-known antigen that has arcane functions. It is still under investigation, but researchers are optimistic about its beneficial effects.

Communication

The immune system communicates through peptides and proteins, secreted by one cell and received by another. These messenger chemicals proceed along the body's systemic pathways.

The messenger substances include cytokines (from *cyto,* "cell" and *kine,* "movement"), proteins that take about four to six hours for the body to manufacture, and polypeptides or neuropeptides, consisting of amino acids, the precursors of proteins. The latter take less time to manufacture and thus are more quickly available.

Endocrine messengers are substances released for a general purpose in a far-off area; *exocrine* messengers are secreted in a tube or "duct" (and into the bile duct); and *paracrine* messengers are local molecules that regulate between two cells in a local area or themselves stimulate other immune activity. Each messenger system is specific as to which cell membrane it fits—it's called the key and lock theory. Part of a messenger fits into the cell's "lock," like a docking lock on a spacecraft, and turns the key. The cell membrane then opens or activates another program or secretes something into the system.

The most amazing thing is that the nerve cells, the immune cells, and the endocrine cells have receptors not only for their own messages but also for those of other systems. The nervous system, for example, has receptors for both the immune and the endocrine messages that are coming in. That's how information is exchanged at the cellular level, and how your immune system can affect your neurological system and vice versa. Thus *illness can cause depression, and depression can cause illness.*

THE IMMUNOLOGIC PROCESS

Assume that a virus or some form of bacterium has gained access to your body, where it has started growing and multiplying. A macrophage engulfs it, processes the proteins on its membranes, and then takes the antigen—which has made the organism unique—and passes it to a helper T cell, which binds it to the macrophage. This union causes the macrophage to release messenger proteins that work to activate quiescent T cells. From them, B cells are stimulated to participate in the response. The B cells will continue secreting antibodies and humoral factors until they are told by suppressor cells that they are no longer needed; then the immune system returns to normal, the invader having been vanquished.

The lymphatics play a vital role in this process. Remember, unless secreted directly into the bloodstream, all the messenger proteins and the intermediary metabolites and toxic waste created by this interaction must be processed through the lymphatics and on into the liver or kidneys. Indeed, many of the immune cells and messenger-producing cells reside in the lymphatic system, and the lymphatic system must be able to get these messengers and immune cells to various parts of the immune system.

If the lymphatic system is slowed down, the initial reaction to the invading organism is severely impaired. The call to alarm cannot be circulated to the cells, their response is delayed or diminished, and the toxins—produced by the interaction of the body with the invading protein—stay in the tissue, evoking a more hyperactive response from the tissue. This in turn causes greater tissue damage, which delays the message for the suppressor T cells to deregulate their activity, thus creating a prolonged overreaction in the tissue. Indeed, an autoimmune process can follow, by which the protein of your *own* body is partially broken down, no longer recognized by the immune cells, and then processed as a foreign protein and treated as such, beginning a long process of inflammatory reaction and autodestruction of your tissues and cells.

THE IMMUNE RESPONSE

The linchpins of nonspecific immunity are the phagocytes, white cells that ingest other cells or microorganisms, debris, and proteins from old and dead cells. Both the phagocytes and the cells of the reticuloendothelial system are deeply involved in any general immune response. They are aided by the "natural killer cells"—nonspecific cyotoxic cells—which destroy malignant or bacterial cells by direct contact.

Complement proteins circulate in the bloodstream and also enhance the immune response. Once they are triggered by a foreign substance or organism, their enzymes digest the edges of the foreign protein and thus attract white cells to the area of inflammation. The complement cascade can be activated by more than just bacteria. In heart-lung surgery, for example, the rough surfaces of the plastic tubes in the heart-lung machine can create a series of reactions by the white cells and complement proteins that causes a total body inflammatory reaction, which can lead to adult respiratory distress syndrome (ARDS), stroke, and renal and/or liver failure. What is normally good for the body can sometimes also become harmful.

LYMPHATICS AS STOREHOUSES

Over and over again during the immune system response, we see the importance of the lymphatics. Besides being a waste removal station for all the body's tissues, they also serve as storehouses for immune cells, such as lymphocytes, and substances that destroy invading organisms and thus act to isolate and neutralize toxins. The lymph nodes filter particulate matter, like bacteria and carbon particles, removing them from circulation. In this way the lymphatic system serves not only as a clearinghouse and filter of the tissue but also as an emergency switchboard where the signal of a messenger substance or alarm from the tissue will mobilize the lymphocytes and the cytokines to react to harmful substances in the circulation.

DETOXIFICATION

Everyone has a level of tolerance to toxicity that cannot be exceeded if good health is to be maintained. We've seen how the immune process works to eliminate toxins. This book is devoted specifically to the care and maintenance of the most important of the immune process delivery systems—the lymphatics—which themselves must be continually detoxified if the entire immune system is to function correctly.

Stagnant or inadequate lymph flow can impair the immune process, as we've seen, but is also associated directly with the onset of many symptoms and illnesses, including arthritis, bursitis in the shoulders, joint stiffness, dry flaking skin, lethargy, depression, and other, more serious diseases like cancer.

A toxic lymphatic system can also lead to hypertension. Dr. William Lee Crowden recommends treating hypertension with dry brushing of the skin for ten minutes daily over the course of three weeks. Use a dry brush with soft vegetable-fiber bristles, and brush the entire body—gently at first, then using firmer strokes—moving the brush toward the middle of the collarbone on each side of the

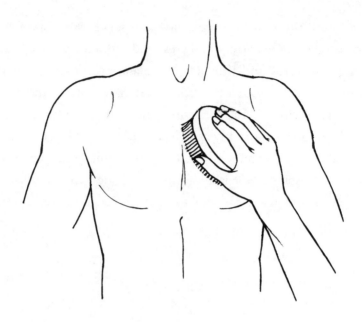

body, since the key lymph drainage sites are located there. Dry brushing helps the skin itself detoxify, invigorates the nervous system, and stimulates lymph drainage.

Since lymph flow depends on muscle contractions and body movements, it follows that exercise, massage, and other compression of the tissue can be of enormous benefit. That's why I've devoted a chapter to exercise and massage. They are as important as diet in maximizing lymphatic flow, and a vital part of the detoxification process.

*   *   *

The immune system must fight its natural enemies, and your body is remarkably equipped to do so. Man-made toxins present more of a problem, for when the human body was originally created and engineered, toxic waste was not around.

In addition, a particular *societal* toxin was not around, one that is not a substance and that stems not from what we manufacture but from the way we act, having profound effects on our physical health and emotional well-being. It is a toxin that has grown more and more virulent with every decade, and there seems little hope that it will grow less dangerous in the new millennium.

It is called stress.

5

Stress

As recently as fifty years ago, the only time we thought of stress was in relation to bridges or buildings. Engineers used the word to refer to the force or pressure exerted on an object; that material changed depending on the resistance it offered to the stress. We laypeople barely had the concept in our brains.

Now, however, stress is part of our everyday vocabulary. "I'm stressed out," we tell our friends. Or "All I get in my job is stress." And it's true. Stress is an increasing factor in our lives. Given the juiced-up pace of American life, the pressures of work (far greater than they were even two decades ago), the desire to "have it all," we are under tremendous pressure. We, as well as bridges, are objects subject to great force.

Our stress comes primarily from change. Its route is from the status quo through chaos to a new (better or worse) place or, as psychologists say, from order to disorder to reorder. External conditions and the temporal qualities of life are constantly changing, and we must change accordingly. Sometimes the stresses are small—a paper due the following day, shopping to be done for the night's meal—and sometimes they are tremendous—the death of a family member, a promotion or a firing, a new relationship or rifts in an old one. As living beings we cannot avoid life, so we must recognize that stress (change) is going to be constantly with us.

It's not stress but how we *respond* to stress that affects our health. Some people thrive in stressful situations; others have a difficult time of it. And all of us are different in what we find stressful.

Stress can be emotional, physical, environmental, or psychological. And stressors can act on our bodies, our minds, our emotions, and our spirits. Yet when it comes to our physical health, stress on any aspect of our being follows the same pathway.

THE NERVOUS SYSTEM'S CHAIN OF COMMUNICATION

The nervous system communicates in two ways: by nerve signals passing between nerve cells and by neuropeptides, molecules of complex amino acids that create a response in the nervous system when secreted. The neuropeptides can stimulate emotions such as fear, pain, sadness, or joy. The seat of these emotions is the hippocampus, that part of the brain connected to the hypothalamus and pituitary gland. When the hippocampus is stimulated, the neurological, endocrine, and immune systems are all activated; all contain receptors for the neuropeptides. The neuropeptides are like telegrams sent to coordinate and allow the body to act in concert. The immune cells and nerve cells, for example "talk" to each other by means of neuropeptides.

These messages are also sent to the endocrine glands, such as the adrenal and thyroid, which are then stimulated to secrete cortisone, epinephrine, and the other hormones vital in the "fight or flight" reaction that the body has built up over millions of years when faced with danger. The clotting system also receives the messages, since if the body is wounded, it must act to stop the bleeding.

Acute stress of any kind focuses on the medulla—the core of the adrenal gland—which releases adrenaline. Chronic stress depletes the cortex, or outer wrapping, of the adrenal gland, which secretes cortisone. Adrenaline increases blood pressure and heart rate and makes the heart work faster—again, for good or ill. Cortisone suppresses the immune system and inflammation and helps regulate the utilization of glucose by the body. Chronic stress exhausts the adrenal gland and sets the body up for a depressed immune system and difficulties in handling the activities of normal life.

The whole reaction to stress is a stimulation of the sympathetic nervous system, which, by nerve conduction to the adrenal glands, increases the secretion of adrenaline and the release of neuropeptides. This, along with increasing adrenaline and cortisone, also speeds up the metabolism of the body. The increased metabolism, in turn, releases free radicals that cause cell damage and destruction.

In other words, an adverse response to stress can damage and eventually kill.

Physical and Psychological Danger

The physical danger our caveman ancestors faced has been replaced by mentally *perceived* danger—psychological danger—but the effect on the body is the same. It is well known that psychological and emotional stress can lead to high blood pressure, chest pain, heart attacks, and death. Recent studies have documented these events and isolated the phenomena that cause them. In the May 1998 issue of the *Journal of the American College of Cardiology,* Dr. Dwaker

Jain of the Yale Medical School reported on his study of 21 patients with coronary heart disease. He subjected them to difficult arithmetic problems and anger recall, then compared them with a group of patients who had been subjected to physical stress through exercise.

Dr. Jain was looking at the ejection fraction of the left ventricle (the percentage of blood that is expelled from the ventricle with each heartbeat). This should be above 55 percent of the total volume of blood in the heart. If the ejection fraction decreases, it is a sign of decreased function of the heart muscle. To his surprise, 43 percent of his patients had a significant change in their ejection fraction, compared with 33 percent of the patients who were exercised. His conclusion: mental stress was at least as potent as physical stress in the exacerbation of heart disease.

The Jain results were complemented by a number of other studies examining stress factors in the overall health of the subject.

- In the August 1999 issue of the *American Journal of Clinical Nutrition,* Dr. Catherine Lefeur showed that mental stress increases triglycerides and LDL and lowers HDL after a meal.
- Researchers at the University of Kuopio, Finland, showed that positive events had a fivefold chance of lowering cholesterol in middle-aged men as compared with negative events, which can raise it.
- Dr. C. M. Stoney of Ohio State University reported in the July 1999 *Life Sciences Journal* that homocysteine levels are elevated in women during psychological stress, even if the women are in perfect health.
- Doctors in the Netherlands demonstrated that when students undertook stressful psychological tasks or academic tests, there was a marked change in their heart rate, blood

pressure, and plasma epinephrine levels. (They found, too, that different postures affected these same indicators. Those who sit for long periods each day without deep breathing and without clearing the lymphatic system keep adrenal mediators and chemical hormones circulating for too long, whereas moving around and exercise can clear them.)

- In June 1999, Dr. Vicki Helgeson, professor of psychology at the Carnegie-Mellon Institute, reported on a study of self-esteem and optimism (the two went hand in hand) in 292 patients who had undergone successful angioplasty. Angioplasty is used to widen an artery; closure means it has narrowed again. In the group that proclaimed the most optimism and self-esteem, the closure rate was 10 percent; the group with the lowest self-esteem had a 30 percent closure rate. Depression, she summarized, was related to heart problems; feelings of joy and happiness promised less chance of cardiac malfunction.

- In a study group of 680 Japanese children watching a provocative TV program called *Pocket Monster,* ionized calcium fell and the pituitary hormone rose, making muscles and nerves more excitable. Those who listened to a quiet program of classical music had no such fluctuation. And this from just a video!

- In the April 1999 *Annals of Medicine,* Dr. A. Appals noted that feelings of exhaustion are not infrequently the first harbinger of a coronary event and that prolonged exposure to stress results in exhaustion. In a study of 30 patients after angioplasty, 15 exhausted and 15 nonexhausted, the level of inflammatory cytokines (proteins expressed by cells to cause an inflammatory reaction in the body) were higher in the exhausted patients and not in the non-exhausted ones.

- Doctor N. Kraus found that only stresses arising from highly valued roles—relating to family, work, or service—would cause health changes. Thus the stressor itself is not important unless it's in an area highly valued by the individual.

- The Department of Surgery in Amsterdam reported an interaction between psychological stressor, neuroendocrine and immunologic processes, and tumor progression. These doctors emphasized that coping mechanisms, even if some of them are negative in nature, are helpful in prolonging a person's life. So is a social network.

- In a study by a group in Oregon, it was shown that breast cancer patients live an average of eighteen months longer if they have group therapy and a social structure of people to talk to.

NATURAL AND PHYSICAL CAUSES OF STRESS

We know that external and environmental events such as earthquakes, war, and hurricanes can trigger arteriosclerotic events. So can the death of a loved one in a natural tragedy such as, ironically, a heart attack.

In fact, in 20 percent of heart attacks, there is a contributing factor that frequently plays a role as a causative agent. This can be a burst of anger, sexual activity, or sudden fear from real or imagined causes. Too much exercise—overexertion—can cause heart failure, even in otherwise healthy individuals. The most vivid example is that of Jim Fixx, whose bestselling *The Complete Book of Running* advocated a daily run of up to 20 miles but who died suddenly in his fifties from following his own regimen. The forty-five-minute brisk walk I advocate is a good deal safer and just as beneficial. (And the warnings on treadmills, StairMasters, and Exercycles to stop exercising when short of breath or feeling fatigued are well worth heeding.)

Among the stressors that can bring early death is bereavement, the "broken heart syndrome." In the United States, over 700,000 people over the age of fifty lose their spouses annually. Of these, 35,000 die during the first year after the spouse's death and, 20 percent or 7,000 of these deaths are directly attributable to the loss of the spouse. There is a profound alteration in cardiovascular and immune response in these patients, so that the mortality rate for the surviving spouse is up to twelve times higher than that of married individuals the same age.

Another disease-producing stressor is social isolation. People living alone without the support of family, friends, or peer groups are at far greater risk of disease than those whose lives are full, no matter at what age.

Job stress is a huge factor in illness, though it is more dissatisfaction with the job than job pressure that is so harmful. In 1971 David Jenkins demonstrated that patients who are under fifty when they have their first heart attack usually have no major risk factors except their jobs or the fact that they live in isolation. Also, the most common period for a heart attack is Monday morning between 8 and 9 A.M., the beginning of the workweek. Dr. Susan Cabasa identified the job qualities that offer protection against morbidity and mortality in the job setting—what she calls the three Cs: (1) control and personal decision making; (2) challenge, a feeling of personal growth and knowledge; (3) commitment, both to the job and to life outside the job. These three attributes improve the chances of avoiding job-induced illness or death.

Your individual feeling about your state of health has a large bearing on how healthy you are. Sociologist Ellen Idler of Rutgers University studied over 2,800 people and got results consistent with five earlier, larger studies involving 23,000 people. The studies concluded that one's own opinion about one's state of health was a better predictor of health than objective factors such as laboratory tests, yearly physical examinations, or even unhealthy behavior such as cigarette smoking. (This is not to say that you should avoid yearly checkups or begin to smoke. People who smoked were twice as likely to die during a given twelve-year period than those who did not. But of the smokers, those who felt they were in bad health were seven time more likely to die than those who said their health was excellent.)

Furthermore, the quality and duration of life you expect plays a part in how well you do. People who say, "My father lived to be ninety years old," often expect a good quality of long life because of it. Similarly, people whose parents died young often expect a short life span—and perhaps their "live fast while you can" attitude helps fulfill this prophecy.

That brain and body are intrinsically linked, and not only in stress-related circumstances, is perhaps shown most vividly in the "nocebo effect" in which negative outcomes result from a harmless pill, the opposite of the "placebo effect." In a British Cancer Group study, a cohort of patients were given placebos but led to believe they were undergoing chemotherapy: 30 percent suffered hair loss, and 50 percent were stricken with nausea and vomiting.

Depression can be an effect of stress or a cause of stress; in either case it is a serious health problem. At the University of Minnesota, a study was conducted of 100 patients going through bone marrow transplants to combat leukemia. The 13 who were diagnosed with major depression had all died within one year. The 87 who were not depressed were all alive two years later. Similarly, Dr. David

..egel showed that women with metastatic breast cancer who worked with a strong support therapy group had an average life expectancy eighteen months greater than those who did not participate in such groups.

Hatred, resentment, bitterness, feelings of unfairness and persecution—all these are causes of stress if they are experienced over protracted periods. All cause significant chemical and hormonal changes in the body; all may well be precursors of disease.

REMEDIES

My overall program, described in Part II, will do much to eliminate unnecessary stress and help you cope with the inevitable stressors life brings to all of us. Still, there are many remedies that have proved particularly helpful in alleviating the effects of stress. Many have to do with the mind, and all are meant to calm, soothe, and balance the frantic pace of our lives with the peace we should bring into all our days.

Spirituality

I use the word *spirituality* here to mean a sense of being part of something greater than oneself so that one's existence transcends present circumstances. I don't necessarily mean a belief in God or even in a Higher Power but rather an extension of obligation and opportunity above and beyond functioning for oneself.

That spirituality is a vital component of health—an idea poohpoohed by the medical establishment as recently as ten years ago—has now been demonstrated in large-scale studies at Duke, Dartmouth, UCLA, the University of California–Berkeley, and even that bastion of traditional medicine, Johns Hopkins. What the

Eastern world has known for thousands of years, the Western world now believes. The beneficial effects of spirituality and prayer have been shown in studies of heart disease, hypertension, stroke, cancers of the uterus and colon, inflammations of the bowel, enteritis, and many other organ systems. Norman Cousins, in his 1979 *Anatomy of an Illness*, described how laughter cured his "incurable" disease; Lawrence LeShan has shown that a positive attitude affects the outcome of cancer; even spontaneous remission has been shown to occur by altering the self-regulatory processes—the positive attitude—of the individual in mind-body experiments. (I'll discuss all this further in Chapter 9, Spirituality.)

We cannot, of course, make ourselves believe in something just because it will benefit our health, but in each of us, I'm convinced, there is a core of spirituality that can be nurtured and made to grow. Perhaps it is enough to believe in the basic goodness and beauty of the world. It's no coincidence that so many ill people find replenishment in nature and are soothed by a forest or the sea.

Meditation

A means of relaxing the body and calming the mind, meditative practices are self-directed approaches to stilling the mind's busyness. They have a long history as part of both Eastern and Western religions, but again, being religious is not essential. Meditation can be quiet contemplation of nature, or the room you sit in, or a thought of the oneness of the universe, or the beauty of the moment.

One common meditative practice is to focus your attention and remove distracting thoughts by repeating a phrase, word, or sound over and over while sitting in a comfortable position. This requires practice, but millions have achieved it and come to rely on it for solace and support. Herbert Benson, a Harvard cardiologist, studied this practice in the late 1960s and concluded that meditation lowered blood cholesterol levels brought on by stress, reduced blood pressure, alleviated anxiety and chronic pain, and improved longevity and the quality of life. He believes meditation is important in combating the inhibition of the immune function and disorders of arousal that arise from overstimulation of the hippocampus.

Mental Imaging

Either with a prompter or guide or through one's own efforts, one enhances physiological processes by imagining the process being desired. For example, one can fight AIDS, if not cure it, through imagery of T cells or decrease stress through imagery of a quiet, peaceful place in your life.

Many studies have shown that mental imagery can bring about significant biochemical and physiological changes. As a health care tool, it can effect thermal and cardiovascular changes and affect the oxygen supplied to the tissue, reflexes of the eye and ear, heart rate, salivation, gastrointestinal activity, blood glucose levels, brain wave alteration, and many other physiological responses. Through mental rehearsal—picturing a situation in your mind—you can relieve anxiety, pain, and the side effects of an intervention. Imaging has successfully relieved the nausea and vomiting associated with chemotherapy, facilitated weight gain in cancer patients, improved immunity—and relieved stress.

Hypnosis

A more controversial means of alleviating stress, hypnosis does not work with everyone, and it is a discipline full of quackery—doctors and psychologists rather than "magicians" should use it as a healing technique. Nevertheless, under deep trance, suggestible patients have been helped enormously, not only in the areas of stress and anxiety but in the treatment of asthma, skin blisters, warts, poison ivy—even the bleeding of hemophiliacs. In one case, my partner, Dr. Paschal Spagna, was asked to do an abdominal resection on a patient who could not have anesthesia because of lung disease. The patient was hypnotized, and the operation was performed. The patient experienced no pain, though he did complain of a sensation of cold when his aorta was cross-clamped. Later the patient was hypnotized whenever he experienced postoperative pain—and the pain disappeared. (And some doctors *still* think there is no connection between body and mind!)

BIOFEEDBACK Techniques of biofeedback teach the voluntary control of autonomic physiological functions, such as brain wave activity, blood pressure, heart rate, and gastrointestinal activity. Yogis over the centuries have been known to slow their heart rates down to six beats a minute and their breathing to a few breaths an hour. My medical school anatomy professor assured me that he personally saw a swami sit in a bathtub and by reverse peristalsis—changing the muscles of the large bowel from expelling to impelling—suck up water from the tub, cleanse his bowel, and expel the water back into a toilet.

Yoga

Yoga performed from twenty minutes to an hour a day improves muscle tone, massages the internal organs, increases blood circulation, allows for deeper breathing and the balancing of the sympathetic and parasympathetic nervous systems, and aids lymphatic flow. We'll discuss yoga more in Chapter 7, for it is a fine tool for maintaining healthy lymphatics. When related specifically to stress reduction, it is a means of relaxation, of slowing down, and, perhaps most important, of regulating the breath—one of the key elements in my overall program. It helps in chest expansion and the ability to hold your breath; it increases the vital capacity and total volume of the lungs. When we're about to go into a particularly stressful situation, we tell ourselves, "Take a deep breath." We can do this without yoga, of course, but yoga helps develop the capacity for breathing, which is the capacity for health.

BALANCE

Balance is a theme I will come back to over and over again; indeed it is the cornerstone of my entire program. And it is particularly vital in the area of stress management.

We've seen how stress, both physical and psychological, can cause disease, though technically it is not the stress that evokes harmful chemicals in our bodies but the reaction to the stressors. The reaction is called emotion, and it is the negative emotions— fear, anger, depression, and hate—that can develop into heart disease, cancer, arthritis, and a host of other chronic degenerative diseases. People who are always depressed, always angry, always afraid, always hating are at as much risk of disease as heavy smokers or heavy drinkers.

On the other hand, positive emotions like joy and love, gratitude and belongingness encourage production of chemicals called endorphins and enkephalins that are healing in nature. One cannot go through life without negative emotions, and one should not go through life without positive ones. It is the balance between the two that we must strive to maintain, a balance based on an awareness of our position in the universe and our relationship with our own being, each other, and all living creatures. Today we seem to be more impressed by human doings than by human beings. The antidote, I believe, is realization of a wisdom outside ourselves that encourages us to be useful and kind and helpful to others. It is there that our happiness lies.

Did you ever notice that sometimes things that are not usually disturbing become particularly irritating, or perhaps things that usually bother us don't seem to matter? This is the interface between the stressor and the emotional reaction. We can try to remove ourselves from the stressor or tell ourselves that we shouldn't be upset, even though we are, but these are generally futile remedies—the stressors keep coming. The physical or emotional environment you're in can add to the pressure as well. For example, if your system is overloaded with difficult tasks and one more irritation is introduced, you'll often overreact by displaying inordinate anger, harbor resentment for your "trials," or bottle up anger that may be difficult to let go of later.

The emotional state that overcomes this and similar problems is called equanimity, commonly also referred to as balance. Balance is the state of being centered, of realizing what's important or permanent and thus evaluating incoming potentially stressful events. It is looking at your life—at the world—as a whole and seeing your reaction to stress in that context. Let's say it's 2 A.M. and your sixteen-year-old daughter isn't home yet. You're frantic with worry until the front door slams, and there she is. Now you're furious and you scream at her, leaving both of you in tears. You've gone through extremes of emotions—love and rage—and the stress is enormous. If only you could step back and parse the situation objectively. Then you'd realize that you're happy she's home and that your anger is self-centered (she made *you* worry), and perhaps you'd realize that a better reaction was possible: talking through your feeling without the rage, without the stress.

This would be regaining psychological balance, but there is also physical, spiritual, and emotional balance. In a greater sense, balance pertains to centering ourselves not only in terms of our reactions but also in terms of our focus. It is, of course, important to be focused when involved in a specific act, whether at work or at home, but to tie up one's life in the single-minded pursuit of a job, an avocation, a dream, or a relationship can be harmful. The workaholic with a neglected family is a typical example of this.

We must balance the time we spend in work, sleep, leisure, physical activity, and spiritual reflection. A well-rounded life will minimize our emotional response to stressors. This is particularly important in negative situations, when an awareness of the world as a whole—the long view as well as the short—can restore equilibrium and perspective.

We can create a positive attitude and deal with negative emotions by:

- Seeking social support
- Laughing often
- Practicing yoga and meditation
- Setting positive goals and making positive affirmations
- Recognizing negative "self-talk" and asking better questions
- Visualizing positive outcomes
- Being optimistic

Balance is vital to wellness. In the program for the health of the lymphatic system—and the body as a whole—that follows, it is not enough to exercise, to diet, to meditate, or to breathe correctly. One must view them all as equally important. All in combination will ensure that the river of life keeps flowing.

PART II

Prevention

To contract a chronic degenerative disease, three conditions must be met:

1. There must be an initiating agent present, a toxin. This could be a trauma, a virus, cholesterol, homocysteine, a bacterium, or some kind of environmental toxin like DDT or heavy metals.
2. There must be a hyperinflammatory response to the oxidative stress caused by the toxin.
3. There must be poor drainage of the toxin so that the toxin stays in contact with the tissue long enough to set up the response.

The last component is what I'm primarily concerned with in this book, for clearance of the toxin is the job of the lymphatics. The smoothly flowing river ensures bodily health. If the lymphatics are clogged, the metabolites that cause toxic reactions stay around and the message proteins that shut off the inflammatory responses in the tissue do not get circulated to the rest of the body, instructing it to produce compounds that will minimize the inflammatory response. It's as simple as that.

When I talk about prevention, I advocate a four-pronged attack.

1. Eliminating or minimizing the toxins
2. Beefing up the body's defense mechanisms with antioxidants and supplements
3. Increasing the lymphatic flow
4. Balancing mind and body—the spiritual, mental, and physical aspects of our being—in a coordinated approach to well-being

This section presents the overall preventive program I recommend. Part III describes how to expand or modify the program in case you already have a disease. But whether you're preventing a disease or the worst of its effects, balance is essential. Diet, breathing, exercise, and stress modification techniques, including meditation, yoga, relaxation, and the careful combination of work and free time are all fine in themselves, but it is the way we balance them that truly accounts for health. I've seen many passionate dieters who do not exercise or who remain workaholics; vitamin nuts who eat a horrific diet; exercise fanatics who light a cigarette with their after-run milkshakes. All of them are at risk.

The Eastern balance of yin and yang, like our own of work and play and rest and exercise, is fundamental to my program and has a vital link to the lymphatics. To my knowledge, this has not been discussed in other health books. So while I discuss each component of a healthy lymphatic system—indeed, a healthy life—separately, it

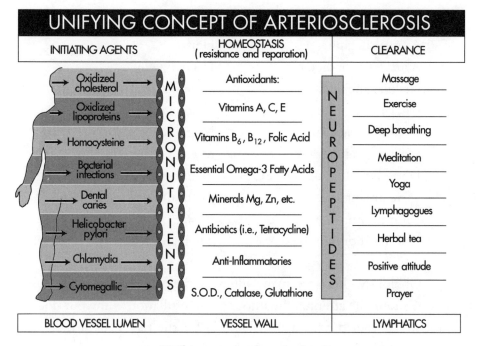

Unifying concept of arteriosclerosis

must be with the reader's knowledge that they are all intertwined. No one element can truly be effective unless it is balanced with the others.

ALTERNATIVE MEDICINE

Mind-body intervention; diet and nutrition; herbal remedies; manual healing methods; chiropractic; energy healing; environmental medicine; all these are "alternatives" to traditional drugs and surgery and can be—often should be—used as adjuncts to them. These methods are incorporated into but not inclusive of the following alternative healing systems:

Acupuncture	Hair analysis
Aroma therapy	Herbs
Ayurvedic medicine	Homeopathy
Cellular therapy	Hypnosis
Chelation	Iridology
Colonic irrigation	Magnetic therapy
Craniosacral therapy	Massage
Dimethylsulfoxide (DMSO) treatment	Naturopathy
	Orthomolecular medicine
Faith healing	Reiki
Folk (traditional) medicine	Therapeutic touch

Obviously, there are many different therapies to consider, and none should be attempted without full consultation with your doctor. What your doctor will evaluate first is the risk/benefit ratio—that is, the risk you take for the benefit you may receive from the therapy. This is patently a key issue, but many alternative systems, *when used in an integrative program,* may have substantial benefits at very little risk, a fact of which many patients are already aware.

In a fascinating recent article in the *Journal of the American Medical Association* Dr. David Eisenberg reported that Americans spent over $27 *billion* in 1997 on alternative therapies, more than is spent out of pocket for specialists, primary care physicians, and hospitalization. Yet perhaps out of guilt, shame, embarrassment, or fear of physician disapproval, more than 50 percent of the people who use alternative systems don't tell their doctors about it. This is a huge mistake, since traditional medications can often interact with or be affected by, say, the micronutrition they are taking.

By now many, though not enough, American doctors are referring patients to alternative therapists, a practice common in Germany, for example, where 95 percent of physicians use herbalists and homeopathists. (Since 1993 a course in herbal medicines has been mandatory in German medical schools.) In the Netherlands, of 600 medical doctors reviewed, 97 percent made referrals to alternative practitioners; in New Zealand, the number was between 70 and 77 percent. In the United Kingdom, 98 percent of the general practitioners and 70 percent of hospital-based doctors routinely refer patients to acupuncture, homeopathy, and hypnosis practitioners.

We're still way behind, partly because of a lack of documentation for efficacy and safety, partly because the practices are not generally taught in U.S. medical schools, and primarily, I suspect, because there is usually no reimbursement by insurance providers.

It's a great shame. Perhaps this book will convince my colleagues that an integrative program is the best means toward optimum recovery and long-lasting health.

6

Diet and Micronutrition

If you had a brand-new Rolls-Royce and filled its gas tank every week with kerosene, people would think you were crazy. But every day those same people fill the most exquisite machine ever devised, the human body, with junk foods and toxins. Our food intake has been so skewed by personal preference ("I eat it because it tastes so good") and depleted by refining, processing, and the exhausting of micronutrients that our bodies are being overloaded with toxins and empty calories while being denied the building blocks for making the enzymes to nullify oxidative stress and aging.

A high-fat, high-protein, low–complex-carbohydrate, low-fiber diet is the American standard. About 45 percent of our calories come from fats, most of which are saturated fats derived from meat and dairy products, although there has been a recent trend to substitute polyunsaturates. The proteins are usually from animal sources, like most of the saturated fats, and the carbohydrates are usually simple ones, such as fructose, glucose, lactose, and sucrose. Refined starches such as potatoes, white pasta, bagels, and white flour are the carbohydrate sources. The acronym for our standard American diet is SAD.

Indeed.

REDUCING FATS IN THE DIET

One antidote for SAD—cutting down on fats and substituting polyunsaturated fats and oils for saturated fats—has created problems of its own. A significant reduction of fat intake seriously limits the intake of essential fatty acids, especially the omega-3s, which are tools for battling degenerative diseases like arteriosclerosis. Reduction of fat intake also reduces caloric intake, and these calories are too often replenished by the addition of simple carbohydrates such as sugar to the food.

Ironically, the significant increase in obesity in the United States over the last decade has come about not because we're ingesting too much fat but because we're substituting sugar for fat. Today 50 percent of Americans are overweight, and nearly 3 million American women are more than 100 pounds above their ideal weight.

As noted previously, unsaturated fats and oils have to be hydrogenated to make them solids at room temperature. Unfortunately, these polyunsaturates are susceptible to oxidation when used in cooking or in packaged foodstuffs such as doughnuts, cookies, and cakes. Their addition to the diet can thus do more harm than good.

THE DIET FOR LYMPHATIC HEALTH

When I advocate a diet program to promote health, fight degenerative disease, and in general lead to physical and spiritual well-being, I approach it in several ways.

The first takes us back to balance. The objective should be to improve ourselves in all areas of our life rather than focus on diet alone. But when it comes to diet, here too balance is the key. It's why I'm so against fad diets, eating the same foods at every meal, or fasting. Yes, I advocate eating little or no meat, cheese, or cake, but there remains a vast panoply of foods that will guarantee variety and enjoyment. We should take the time to savor our meals, to be cognizant of the taste and texture of what we eat, the benefits each mouthful gives us, and the wonderful blessings we get from eating. It's important to tie in our spiritual, mental, and physical environment by being cognizant of the time and love that went into the preparation of the food and by relaxing during the meal so that it is not colored by negative emotions like anger or anxiety. Also, we should take our *time*. When we gulp down our meals, we deny ourselves pleasure, and what good is life without pleasure?

Second, we should decrease or eliminate the toxins in our foods. For most people, a healthy diet would consist of a high–complex-carbohydrate meal with about 20 percent fat and 15 to 20 percent protein. Until recently, however, the SAD was about 50 percent fat, 20 percent protein, and 30 percent mostly simple carbohydrates. As noted, the low-fat diet of recent years has changed the percentages, but it's meant that our sugar consumption has grown to about 170 pounds per person per year. Substitution of artificial sweeteners is no solution. They can be carcinogenic.

And our salt consumption is up to almost 9 grams a day, most of it hidden in the processed foods and drink we consume on a daily basis. Salt can cause hypertension and its attendant problems. Sugar has been linked to cancer, heart disease, and a variety of infections. It has been shown to elevate the triglycerides, lower HDL, decrease the white cell immune response, and generally cause great bodily debilitation.

The simplest way to avoid these toxins is by reading labels and not buying foods high in fat, sugar, or salt. Another way is to follow the diet proposed in this book with its concomitant recipes, remembering that a small percentage of people—perhaps 5 to 10 percent—really need a higher fat and protein intake because of their insulin resistance. Specialty diets, like the Zone Diet and the Sugar Buster Diet and even the Atkins Diet, are popular because people do lose weight with them even though they are high in fat and protein. However, the long-term effects of continued ingestion of saturated fats and casein from milk products are of course not seen until many years after the diet has been initiated, and there is no way of tallying these effects into the immediate benefits.

Third, I advocate following several rules of thumb in looking at what to eat or prepare. These are general and certainly don't apply to 100 percent of the population, but they're a good starting point and should be remembered.

1. Avoid all white foods—sugar, white flour products such as white bread, bagels, and pasta, ice cream, eggs, cheese, and milk products. The vast majority of them are processed foods or dairy products, high in fat and cholesterol. Intake should be totally elim- inated or reduced to a minimum because processed foods contain empty calories; that is, where the vitamins and minerals have been removed and the intake is pure simple carbohydrates or fats. If you must eat yogurt, milk, ice cream, or cheese, switch to low-fat or fat- free products. It's important to get calcium to avoid osteoporosis, but the fat and protein in dairy products can leach calcium out of the body into the bowel. It's far better to use calcium supplements and to substitute soy milk or rice milk for cow's milk.

2. Three times a week, eat a dinner of plants only. In these meals there should be no seafood, meat, chicken, or dairy products. Eat- ing more vegetables and fruits—the plant foods—can reduce the risk of cancer of the colon, stomach, mouth, throat, esophagus,

lungs, pancreas, and bladder, as well as lessening the risk of heart disease and stroke. The proteins can be supplied by beans, soybeans, lentils, tofu, and stir-fried vegetables.

3. Don't eat fatty meats or ground beef. In ground beef, the fat is mixed in with the meat and there is no way it can be separated out; the percentage of fat in ground beef is much higher than in lean meat with the fat cut away from it. In addition to the problem of fat, many animals are fed hormones to "beef them up" and are also often on antibiotics as a secondary effect of the hormones.

There is growing evidence suggesting that all meats, even lean red meats, can increase the risk of colon and prostatic cancer, so if you can stay away from them altogether, it's to your health benefit. Red meats are high in saturated fats, the fats that cause cancer and heart disease and elevate your LDL while lowering your HDL. And poultry has almost as much cholesterol as red meat, even if you cut away its fat. My general recommendation is to eat meat as infrequently as possible. If you must eat it, cut it into small pieces and disperse it among vegetables, as in stir-fried or Chinese food. In this way you can get the flavor of the meat without the overload of toxins that comes with it. By the way, a wonderful substitute for hamburger is a veggie burger or tofu burger. Another meat substitute is seitan, which can be cooked to taste like beef or ham. If you're cooking spaghetti sauce, you can prepare soy sausages or soy meatballs instead of their meat equivalents. If you refrigerate the sauce, the fat will rise to the top where you can easily skim it off and end up with a meat-free, fat-free sauce that's as good or better than the "real thing."

4. The soybean is one of the very few plants that are a complete source of protein. It is rich in amino acids and vitamins A, E, K, and some Bs, as well as being low in saturated fats. Substitute soy for meat, and your diet will be far more healthy.

5. Make all your snacks fruits and vegetables. If you eat at least

five to nine servings a day, you'll be taking in the micronutrition of folic acid, potassium, B vitamins, phytochemicals, and fiber that helps reduce heart disease, cancer, and stroke. Keep a bag of peeled baby carrots on your desk, or peel a grapefruit, orange, or tangerine; try any of the delicious types of apples available today; keep a bowl of fresh fruit salad in the refrigerator. My only caveat is that you wash the fruits and vegetables carefully before you eat them (many come from places that don't have the strict pesticide laws we do). Furthermore, it's better if you buy organic vegetables and fruits, though they're expensive. Considerable experimentation is going on now with genetically manipulated fruits and vegetables, but we don't yet know the long-term effects after ingestion—another reason to stick to the organically grown kind, at least for the moment.

6. Avoid pizza and other processed cheese foods. Cheese is high in saturated fats and cholesterol and very high in sodium (about 200 milligrams per pizza slice, to say nothing of its 800 calories). If you eat pizza at all, make sure it's only once a month or so—and try to eat the kind made with low-oil, low-fat cheese.

7. Use whole grains. They are high in fiber and micronutrients that are often depleted from our highly processed food chain. Oatmeal makes a great breakfast, and a high-fiber program in general is always beneficial.

8. Keep alcohol to a minimum. Always choose one or two glasses of red wine instead of hard liquor because with the wine you'll derive the benefit of the antioxidants in the red grape (a benefit, of course, that you can also get from grape juice). Women increase the risk of breast cancer when they drink, and large amounts of alcohol—over three or four drinks a day—can lead to heart disease.

9. Don't overload on sweets. The average 12-ounce soft drink, for example, has 160 empty calories and no fiber, minerals, vitamins, or antioxidants.

10. Substitute olive oil for butter or margarine, and spray your cooking pans with olive or canola oil. If you do use margarine, read the label carefully before you buy, since they may contain trans-fats and polyunsaturates that, when heated, break down and become highly oxidized. As I've noted, unsaturated oils such as corn oil should be avoided not only because of trans-fats but because they are labile and will certainly cause oxidative stress when heated.

11. Cut down on sodium by going easy on prepared or refined food. More than 75 percent of the sodium we ingest comes from processed foods, so as much as possible start everything from scratch. Steam your vegetables, and skip commercial salad dressing, instead mixing your own vinegar, garlic, and mustard with some olive oil. Use lemon juice and, in place of mayonnaise, Vegennaise, a tofu mix that contains no dairy products and hence no cholesterol.

12. Drink 8 to 10 glasses of water a day. Water flushes out the system and is the body's natural lubricant.

13. Drink 1 to 2 cups of tea a day. Green tea contains the polyphenols that enhance the immune system and fight cancer and heart disease. But black tea is also effective. New studies have shown that "white" tea may be even more effective than green tea as an antioxidant. A recent study of 3,454 people in the Netherlands found that those who drank tea daily lowered their risk of severe aortic arteriosclerosis by 46 percent. (Tea's protective effect was more evident in women than in men, though no one as yet knows why.)

14. Cold-water fish make a good protein meal, especially tuna, salmon, mackerel, and halibut, which are a great source of omega-3, an essential fatty acid. Shrimp and lobster can also be eaten occasionally because although they are high in cholesterol, they are also rich in protein and essential fatty acids, including omega-3. Also, some of the cholesterol, though not all, is in the form of phytos-

terol, which can actually block cholesterol absorption in the gut. But it's worth repeating here that you should avoid older large fish such as swordfish or shark because of the amount of heavy metal the fish are forced to ingest, since toxins are being pumped into our oceans at an alarming rate. However, young ocean tuna and salmon, like their freshwater brethren, are fine sources of protein and omega-3 fatty acids.

If you're a vegetarian like Janie and don't want to eat fish, consider flaxseed oil and purslane, a weedlike vegetable eaten extensively in the Middle East and eastern Mediterranean countries. This is a delicious leafy plant, high in omega-3 fatty acids, that can be used in salad and many other ways.

WHY A NEW PYRAMID?

The USDA Food Pyramid was designed in an attempt to illustrate what foods should be included in a healthful diet and how much of these foods should be eaten. Unfortunately, this pyramid makes no distinction between whole grains and refined grains, or between whole grain products and processed or refined grain products. White flour breads and bagels, white rice, white pasta, and refined and processed cereals could theoretically compose the basis of this diet instead of whole grains such as whole wheat, barley, and oats, brown rice, whole wheat pasta and oatmeal, or whole grain cold cereals. Numerous studies have shown fiber's protective role in cardiovascular disease. The *American Journal of Epidemiology* published a study on more than 11,000 men and women that showed that women consuming the highest amounts of fiber had the lowest risk of cardiovascular disease. (High-fiber foods are also plentiful in antioxidants and folate.)

In the USDA Food Pyramid, health-supporting beans and

legumes are grouped with meat, poultry, cheese, and dairy, which are high in cholesterol and saturated fat, not to mention the addition of growth hormones and antibiotics. Milk, yogurt, and cheese are not specified as full fat or skim. Fats and oils at the top of the pyramid are not broken down into "good fats" (essential fatty acids, nondamaged polyunsaturates, and monounsaturated) or "bad fats" (butter, lard, damaged processed oils, and trans-fats). This pyramid suggests that one could have white flour bagels with high-fat cream cheese, white rice, white pasta, full-fat cheese, milk and yogurt, meat, chicken, and eggs regularly, with lard, butter, and heat-treated and chemically processed vegetable oils (used sparingly).

THE LEMOLE PYRAMIDS

Dr. William Castelli of the Framingham Heart Study stated, "Vegetarians have the best diet. They have the lowest rates of coronary disease of any group in the country." The Lemole Pyramids represent a plant-based, whole-food, health-supporting diet, taking the best from both the Mediterranean and Asian diets. This plan is high in fiber, nutrient-dense foods, and essential fatty acids and low in saturated fats, cholesterol, and sugar. It does not include meat, damaged oils, trans-fats, and processed "empty foods." Fish is permitted, because fish and fish oils have been shown to reduce the risk of cardiovascular disease and appear beneficial in preventing heart attacks as well as graft patency after intervention.

Carbohydrates in the Diet

Confusion has developed regarding carbohydrates. Once the darling of dieters and athletes, unspecified carbohydrates were supposedly the basis of a "healthful diet." The message was "push the carbs." Unfortunately the carbs being pushed were *simple* carbohydrates—white processed flour in breads, bagels, pasta, and white rice. Then "insulin resistance" and "syndrome X" became hot topics. Now *carbohydrate* has become a dirty word—and the message of the moment has become "push the protein." Americans already consume excessive amounts of protein. Research indicates that diets high in protein, especially animal protein, cause calcium to be lost in the urine. The more protein consumed, the more calcium is excreted. Research has also shown that high protein intake contributes to kidney disease, putting chronic overload on the body's filtering system. Osteoporosis and kidney failure are common diseases. In a vegetarian or semivegetarian diet, protein is more than adequately supplied by soy, other legumes, beans, whole grains, and fish if included.

Notes on Food Pyramids

WHOLE GRAIN GROUP: At least five servings daily. Whole grains (rice, barley, wheat, oats, etc.) and their whole grain products (whole grain breads, whole grain cereals, both hot and cold, and whole wheat pasta).

VEGETABLE GROUP: At least four servings daily of fresh vegetables. Eat freely and without restrictions unless individual restriction (e.g., cruciferous vegetables and thyroid disease). Include crucifers (broccoli, cabbage), orange and yellows (sweet potatoes, squash), dark leafy greens, seaweed, onions, garlic, and ginger.

FRUIT GROUP: At least three servings daily. Eat freely and without restrictions unless individual restriction (e.g., high triglycerides and diabetes). Include citrus, apples, berries, tropicals (mangoes, papayas), melon, and bananas.

NOTE: While vegetable and fruit juices are excellent, in general it is best to eat the whole fresh fruit or vegetable for increased fiber. This way, even if the fruit or vegetable has a high glycemic index (carrots and potatoes), its fiber assures slow release of sugar.

LEGUMES: At least two to three servings daily. Beans, lentils, peas, soy and soy products, edamame (steamed soy beans), tofu, tempeh, miso, soy hot dogs, burgers, sausage, etc.

UNPROCESSED NUTS AND SEEDS: Small amounts daily (handful).

FISH: Fish and fish oils reduce the risk of cardiovascular disease. Northern cold-water fatty fish—salmon, cod, tuna, herring, sardines, etc.

VEGETABLE OILS: Flaxseed and extra-virgin olive oil. Never heat flaxseed oil. Also, use canola oil for baking and cooking. Use only cold-pressed oil and only in small amounts.

EGGS: Several weekly if desired when cholesterol levels are normal.

The Lemole Beverage Pyramid

Filtered or spring water should be the basic liquid of a health-supporting diet. Green and white tea appear in studies to lower the risk of cardiovascular disease by reducing total cholesterol levels and LDL cholesterol levels. Green tea does contain caffeine and if 6 to 10 cups (as in some studies) are consumed daily, decaffeinated tea is recommended.

Fresh vegetable juices are excellent as are fresh fruit juices

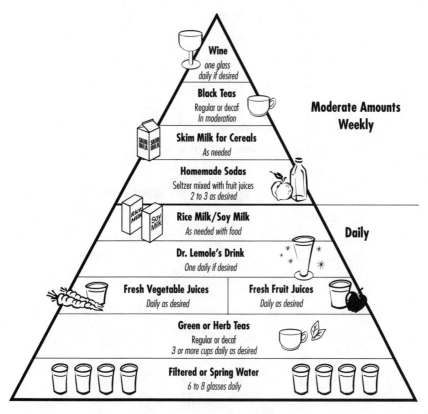

The Lemole beverage pyramid

(except for people with diabetes and high triglycerides). Dr. Lemole's Drink is a powerhouse of nutrition, fiber, and essential fatty acids in a delicious drink—a good breakfast for people in a hurry.

Rice and soy milk are healthful substitutes for milk. Homemade sodas are refreshing without the caffeine, colors, phosphates, sodium, and extra sugar or artificial sweeteners found in soft drinks. Skim-milk products are acceptable if tolerated well. Black teas should be consumed with moderation. Wine, especially red wine, appears to have health benefits (pycnogenol antioxidants) and if desired may be taken in moderation (1 glass a day).

• DR. LEMOLE'S DRINK •

1½ cups fruit juice or soy milk

1 banana (other fruits may be added; peaches and
   kiwis are good)

1 tablespoon flaxseed oil

1 tablespoon powdered vitamin and mineral
   supplements

1 tablespoon green powder from vegetables and
   fruits

1 teaspoon psyllium seed husks (may be gradually
   increased to 1 tablespoon)

1 scoop soy powder

OPTIONAL

2 teaspoons wheat germ

1 tablespoon nutritional yeast

1 tablespoon PC55 phosphatidyl choline

1 tablespoon ground flax seeds (may be used instead
   of flaxseed oil)

Mix all ingredients in a blender, and blend for 30 seconds.

In summary, the most beneficial diet for the majority of patients is
a high complex-carbohydrate diet, which consists of the following:

- Approximately 60 percent to 70 percent complex carbohydrates with little or no sugars and simple starches.
- 15 to 20 percent proteins, mostly from cold-water fish,
  soybeans, lean meats, and beans.
- 15 to 20 percent fat, primarily unsaturated fat found in
  fish, flaxseed oil, monounsaturated olive oil, and canola oil.
- Less than 5 percent saturated fats

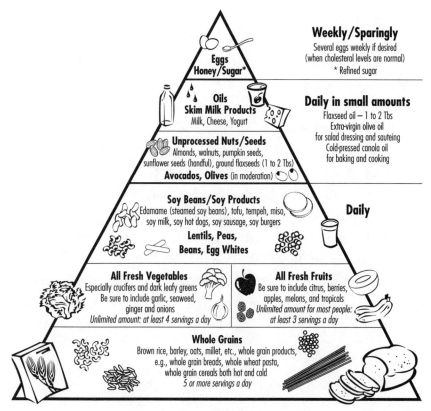

The Lemole vegetarian diet pyramid

- 3 to 5 percent EFAs, primarily omega-3s and some omega-6s derived from fish, flaxseed oil, etc.

This diet decreases levels of cholesterol, LDL, homocysteine, and adipose tissue while increasing EFAs. It also spares calcium and magnesium, which protect against osteoporosis, hypertension, arrhythmia, and other chronic degenerative diseases. A small percentage of patients who may not respond favorably to this diet will need their protein and fat increased at the expense of carbohydrates to control cholesterol, triglycerides, and sugar. It is recommended to get a baseline lipid profile and blood sugar before initiating patients on this high complex-carbohydrate diet for eight weeks, and repeat the lipid and sugar profiles. If these are still elevated, then one should consider changing to a higher protein diet or adding supplements to lower lipids; and only as a last resort, using cholesterol-lowering drugs.

In the United States we've seen a 30-percent reduction in mortality from arteriosclerosis in the last twenty-five years, possibly due to many factors, including diet, better blood pressure control, smoking cessation, increased physical activity and health awareness, along with technological advances in cardiac surgery, interventional cardiology, and medications. Often overlooked as another reason for the decrease in heart disease is the fact that more than 100 million citizens in the United States take vitamin supplements and our foods now have added micronutrients, especially vitamin B_6 and folic acid.

MICRONUTRIENTS

When humans first appeared on earth, they found no industry, no pollution, no pesticides, and few contaminants in the food they hunted and gathered. Even as recently as ninety years ago, our food was relatively pure and we did not need to supplement it with micronutrients. Nature supplied them in the food itself.

But recently, changes in fertilizers, pesticides, and methods of harvesting and preserving food stock by the agro-industry have seriously compromised the natural micronutrients. Cattle and poultry producers have significantly changed feed patterns, which has increased the saturated fats and decreased the essential fatty acids in our livestock. Introduction of antibiotics and growth hormones has contributed to antibiotic-resistant bacteria and B complex vitamin deficiencies. The creation of trans-fats has played a major role in disease. Food suppliers are more concerned about price, shelf life, and visual presentation (those red apples virtually *shine*) than they are about health, which has a negative impact on the micronutrients supplied by their products.

There is good evidence that a large segment of the population is deficient in significant amounts of micronutrients such as magnesium, CoQ_{10}, essential fatty acids, and B vitamins. Among other things, these are the prerequisites for optimum recovery after cardiac intervention, which is why I emphasize them so strongly—I've seen the effects that transpire when micronutrients are depleted. Several studies have shown that a majority of elderly patients are deficient in magnesium, leading to hypertension, arrhythmias, vascular spasm, and activation of the hyperthrombotic state. Similarly, CoQ_{10} can be depleted by the statin drugs, beta-blockers, phenothiazine, vitamin B_6 deficiency, and doxorubicin hydrochloride (Adriamycin), but CoQ_{10} and magnesium are essential to the oxidative process and respiratory reactions in the mitochondria that supply energy to the body.

It is obviously essential, then, that any cardiac patient—and particularly elderly ones—receive supplementary micronutrients. The RDA for normal, healthy adults are woefully inadequate for cardiac patients because of the deficiencies caused by cardiac medications. I think *everyone* should follow instead the optimal daily intake (ODI) recommendations found in the *Real Vitamin & Mineral Book* by Shari Lieberman, Ph.D.

A good example of the difference between the RDA and the ODI can be seen in the recommended amount of vitamin E. In the RDA, it is 10 international units (IU). Yet studies including the Nurses Study and the Physician Study published in the *New England Journal of Medicine* recommended dosages at the level of 400 to 1,200 IU a day to reduce the risk of heart disease and heart attacks.

I'll provide a micronutritional program specifically geared to cardiac patients later in the book. But in general my micronutritional recommendations are five-pronged:

1. Antioxidants: the vitamins A, C, and E, which help burn up or neutralize the free radical oxidative stress that comes with physical and mental stress and aging
2. Minerals: selenium, magnesium, calcium, and zinc, which act as catalysts in the enzymatic processes that are necessary to neutralize the oxidative stress in our bodies
3. Essential fatty acids: omega-3 and omega-6, which decrease the inflammatory response in our bodies and allow for less inflammatory reaction in the arterial wall (In arthritic patients, coronary patients, and some cancer patients, adding fatty acids will reduce the effects of these diseases.)
4. CoQ_{10}: a compound essential for life since it is used by every cell involved in metabolism (After the age of fifty especially if patients are on statin drugs, CoQ_{10} is seriously depleted and replacements are necessary.)
5. B complex: for carbohydrate, protein, and fat metabolism

Dosages for all micronutrients are listed in my specific diet programs in Part III.

HERBS

People have been using herbs for cooking and to treat illness for thousands of years. Indeed, herbs as remedies are depicted in Egyptian tomb paintings, and papyrus documents provide the earliest written medical prescriptions for the use of onions and garlic. Adding herbs to your diet will not only improve the flavor of the food you eat but add important nutrients and micronutrients to your diet.

But remember: The drug industry started by selling "natural remedies"—I think of quinine from the cinchona tree and digitalis from foxglove—and you should be wary of taking herbs unless you know the strength of the doses, since overuse can cause some toxicity. Also, many of these herbs come from third world countries and may be contaminated with metals or sprays from the country of origin; they're not reliably regulated when they're brought into the States. Make sure you buy your natural herb supplements from a reliable company with a good long reputation and a history of fine products.

And now it's time to eat.

FOURTEEN-DAY DIET

This fourteen-day diet is in fact one basic high complex-carbohydrate program meant to jump-start my entire fitness plan. To lose weight, decrease or eliminate the whole grain bread, pasta, and potato dishes. *Also, do not use the recipes marked with an asterisk; these are higher in fats.* If you want a high-protein diet, concentrate on the fish and soy recipes. The point is not to follow the diets slavishly, but to adapt them to your own needs.

BREAKFAST SUGGESTIONS

1. Oliver's Oatmeal—old-fashioned oatmeal with sunflower seeds, chopped walnuts, and dried cranberries
   1% rice or soy milk
   Honey or sugar in moderation
   ½ grapefruit

2. 1 boiled egg (DHA enhanced, if possible)
   2 slices soy Canadian bacon (Yves)
   1 slice seven-grain bread, toasted if desired (with all-fruit spread optional)
   Fresh carrot juice

3. Flax waffles (Lifestream) with blueberries and maple syrup
   Soy sausage (Gimme Lean)
   Sliced papaya

4. Japanese Breakfast
   Miso Soup (page 136)
   Steamed rice
   Seaweed salad

Small piece of broiled salmon with light soy sauce
Green tea

5. Shredded wheat
   1% rice soy milk
   Sliced banana
   Freshly squeezed orange juice
   Handful of raw almonds

6. Magic Drink or Cool Green Magic Drink (pages 157, 158)

7. Poached egg (DHA enhanced if possible) on seven-grain bread
   Prunes stewed in tea and lemon slices

8. Smoked salmon on whole grain bagel, toasted if desired
   Nonfat or low-fat cream cheese, to spread lightly
   Sliced sweet onions and tomatoes, capers, and lemon
   Tomato juice

9. Tofu Scramble* (page 143)
   Sprouted grain toast (with all-fruit spread, if desired)
   Fresh grapefruit slices

10. Banana nut bread muffin
    Low-fat or nonfat organic yogurt
    Sliced fresh fruit assortment

11. Soy burger (Boca) or grain burger (Garden) topped with
    melted soy cheese (pepper jack, mozzarella, or American)
    1 slice tomato
    1 slice seven-grain bread, toasted if desired

12. Soy Flax Shake (page 156)

13. Less the Yolk Omelet (page 142) or One to Three Omelet
    (page 142)

Rosemary Breakfast Potatoes (page 143)
Melon slices

14. All-Bran Buds Cereal (13 grams fiber)
    1% rice or soy milk
    Berries or banana
    Freshly squeezed orange juice.

LUNCH SUGGESTIONS

1. Uncream of Carrot and Ginger soup (page 137)
   Daphne's Baked Tofu Sandwich (page 134)
   Fruit juice soda

2. Harry's Hummus* (page 126)
   Pita bread for scooping
   Chopped Greek Salad* (page 129)
   Cucumber Yogurt Raita (page 155)
   Grapes

3. Soy (Boca) or grain (Garden) burger
   Toasted whole grain bread
   1 tablespoon grapeseed oil, Vegenaise, and ketchup, if desired
   Lettuce, tomato, onion, pickle
   French Unfries (page 154)
   Apple

4. Pasta and Bean Soup (page 138)
   Arugula salad drizzled with extra-virgin olive oil and a squeeze
      of fresh lemon juice; top with shavings of imported Parme-
      san cheese
   Melon slices

5. Shrimp salad using Vegenaise with avocado on a bed of greens
     and beans with Lemon Vinaigrette (page 132)
   Baked or fresh apple

6. Zoe's Split Pea Soup (page 139)
   Tuna salad using Vegenaise on romaine lettuce
   Pear

7. Blue Bell Inn Lentil Salad (page 127) on baby greens
   Apple

8. *Japanese Lunch*
   Edamame (page 126)
   Miso Soup (page 136)
   Seaweed salad (Asian store)
   Fresh pineapple
   Green tea

9. The Compassionate Chef's Salad (page 128)
   Sliced mango with blackberries

10. Pita Pizza—Sienna or Margapita (page 136)

11. Michael's Chickpea Salad or Sandwich (page 131)
    Carrot strips
    Handful of raw sunflower seeds and walnuts

12. Good Friday Soup (page 138)
    White Bean and Tuna Salad (page 128) on spring greens
    Clementines or orange

13. Tofu hot dog (Yves)
    Whole grain hot dog bun (Amarillo), chopped onions,
      sauerkraut, mustard, and ketchup, as desired

French Unfries (page 154)
Fruit-juice Popsicles

14. Mushroom Barley and Kale Soup (page 140)
    Sardines on seven-grain toast
    Sliced pineapple and strawberries

DINNER SUGGESTIONS

1. Festive Salmon Roll* (page 147)
   Steamed asparagus with chopped onion and tomato
   Rosemary Breakfast Potatoes (page 143)
   Sliced papaya

2. *Summer Supper*
   Fast pasta with Fresh Tomato Sauce (page 150)
   Garden salad with fresh herb vinaigrette
   Watermelon or any fruit-juice popsicles

3. Charlie's Tomato Sauce (page 150) with "meat balls" (page 149) and spaghetti*
   Broccoli Baobabs* (page 153)
   Grapes

4. Whole steamed or boiled artichoke with lemon or balsamic vinaigrette (page 132)
   Sweet red roasted peppers (jar) or home-made with anchovies
   White bean and celery salad; drizzle with a little extra-virgin olive oil and a little vinegar over both
   Tropical fruits sliced

5. Stuffed Acorn Squash (page 154)
   Mixed salad—greens, tomato, cucumber, onion, carrots, creamy
      Italian dressing

6. Seared Tuna (page 146)
   Christopher's Rice (page 152)
   Asian Slaw (page 132)
   Fresh fruit sorbet

7. *Mexican Feast*
   Refried Bean Roll-ups (page 135)
   Spanish Rice
   Salsa (page 125) and Bumby Guacamole* (page 125)
   Limeade—fresh lime juice with sparkling water
   Melon

8. *Simplicity Supper*
   Large baked white or sweet potato topped with nonfat sour
      cream
   Spinach salad with citrus dressing and veggie bacon bits
      (Lightlife)
   When potato skin is empty, use as a pita and fill with salad
   Granny Smith apple

9. *Midsummer Supper*
   Baked or grilled salmon filets with Christophers' Marinade
      (page 151)
   Sliced beets with sautéed beet greens
   Corn on the cob
   Sliced tomatoes, cucumbers, onions with balsamic vinaigrette
   Sliced peaches

10. Jerry's Angel Hair Pasta (page 148)
    Crusty rustic or peasant bread
    Caesar Salad* (page 130)
    Sliced oranges

11. Portuguese Baked Cod with Rice (page 144)
    Lima beans and corn
    Green salad with olive oil, vinegar, and oregano
    Sliced apples and grapes

12. Seafood Corn Chowder (page 140)
    Green salad with shiitake mushrooms
    Kiwis and strawberries

13. Don't Worry Curry (page 151)
    Pan-seared tofu
    Steamed brown rice with ponzu sauce (Eden)
    Daddy's rice pudding

14. Portland Country Club's Saké-Glazed Sea Bass (page 146)
    Cucumber avocado roll
    Steamed white or brown rice
    Salad of chopped Asian greens, Chinese cabbage, etc., with
        ginger dressing
    Green tea

15. Scallops, Shrimp, and Clams over Udon with Spicy Asian
        Sauce (page 155)
    Salad with Asian vinaigrette
    Fresh fruit sorbet

RECIPES

• SALSA •

4 large tomatoes, chopped
1 sweet onion, chopped
1 to 2 garlic cloves, pressed or minced
½ cup chopped fresh cilantro leaves
2 tablespoons fresh lime juice
2 fresh jalapeño peppers, sliced, or if too hot, use
    canned chili peppers
Salt and pepper to taste

If a chunky salsa is desired, chop all ingredients by hand and mix together in a bowl. If a smoother salsa is desired, put in food processor until blended. Adjust seasoning.

MAKES ABOUT 2 CUPS

• BUMBY GUACAMOLE* •

4 ripe avocados, peeled and pitted
1 red onion, chopped very fine
1 large tomato, chopped
4 tablespoons fresh cilantro, chopped fine
Hot chiles or 1 jalapeño pepper if desired or hot
    pepper sauce to taste
⅓ cup fresh lime or lemon juice
2 teaspoons ground cumin
Salt and pepper to taste

Mash avocado with a fork. Add remaining ingredients. Adjust desired hotness and seasoning. Cover lightly with plastic wrap and let flavors marry for at least an hour.

MAKES ABOUT 1½ CUPS

• HARRY'S HUMMUS* •

2 cups chick peas (canned or cooked)
1 tablespoon tahini (sesame seed paste)
2 to 3 cloves of garlic—pressed or minced
1 tablespoon extra-virgin olive oil
Juice of 1 large lemon
Salt and pepper to taste
Paprika
Chopped parsley

In a mixer or blender, purée all ingredients except paprika and parsley until smooth. Put in a bowl. Sprinkle with paprika and chopped parsley. Serve at room temperature or chilled as a dip for pita bread.

MAKES ABOUT 2 CUPS

• EDAMAME •

These soybeans in the pod are found in the freezer section. Boil or steam following package directions.

• BLUE BELL INN LENTIL SALAD •

Through the kindness of Chef John Lamprecht

2 cups French green lentils
5 tablespoons vegetarian chicken broth powder
5 cups water
1 small onion, coarsely chopped
1 stalk celery, coarsely chopped
¼ bunch flat-leaf parsley, coarsely chopped
¼ cup tarragon vinegar
1 cup light olive oil
Salt and pepper
Finely chopped onion
Hot sauce

Wash lentils and pick out any debris. Drain lentils and place in pot. Mix the broth powder and water and add to the lentils. Cover and let them soak for 1 hour. Place onion, celery, and parsley in a cheesecloth bag. Add to the lentils and stock. Bring lentils to a boil. Lower to a simmer and cook for 10 minutes or until tender. Drain lentils and let cool.

Make a vinaigrette using the tarragon vinegar, olive oil, salt, and pepper. Whisk together thoroughly. Add to the lentils and toss together.

Serve with finely chopped onion and hot pepper infusion or Louisiana Hot sauce.

SERVES 4

• THE COMPASSIONATE CHEF'S SALAD •

1 head romaine lettuce

1 head leaf or Bibb lettuce

1 green or red bell pepper, cored, seeded, and sliced
 into rings

1 tomato, sliced

1 cucumber, sliced

1 red onion, sliced

2 stalks celery, finely chopped

6 slices soy cheese (Mozzarella, American, or Pepper
 Jack) cut into strips

6 slices soy ham, cut into strips

6 slices soy turkey, cut into strips

OPTIONAL

2 hard-boiled eggs (sliced with or without yolks)

4 radishes, sliced

8 olives

*Arrange artfully in a salad bowl and dress with commercial or homemade
mustard vinaigrette.*

SERVES 4

• WHITE BEAN AND TUNA SALAD •

3 cups canned cannellini beans, drained and rinsed

2 cans albacore tuna in spring water, well separated
 with fork

1 sweet onion, finely chopped

3 stalks celery, finely chopped

¼ cup extra-virgin olive oil

2 tablespoons red wine vinegar

Salt and freshly ground pepper

3 tablespoons chopped fresh parsley

1 tablespoon chopped fresh basil

Put rinsed beans in a large serving bowl. Add tuna, onion, and celery. In a small bowl whisk oil and vinegar together and drizzle over bean and tuna mixture. Season with salt and freshly ground pepper to taste. Sprinkle with parsley and basil. Gently toss again.

SERVES 4 TO 6

• CHOPPED GREEK SALAD* •

1 clove garlic, minced

4 tablespoons extra-virgin olive oil

1 head romaine lettuce

2 cucumbers, peeled and chopped

2 tomatoes, chopped

1 red onion, chopped

1 green bell pepper, chopped

12 kalamata olives

6 ounces feta cheese, cut into cubes

1 tablespoon fresh lemon juice

1 tablespoon red wine vinegar

Salt and finely ground pepper to taste

Press or mince garlic and add to olive oil. Chop the lettuce into bite-size pieces. Combine lettuce, cucumber, tomatoes, onions, and green pepper in a salad bowl. Add olives and cheese, dress with oil, lemon juice, and red wine vinegar. Season with salt and black pepper to taste.

SERVES 4

• CAESAR SALAD* •

1 clove garlic
½ can anchovies
4 tablespoons olive oil
4 tablespoons canola oil
Juice of 1 lemon
Dash of Worcestershire sauce (Lea & Perrins or
   vegetarian)
¼ teaspoon dry mustard
1 head romaine lettuce
1 cup croutons (homemade with/whole-wheat
   bread)
Parmesan cheese or (better) soy Parmesan cheese

Crush garlic and anchovies with a fork in a salad bowl. Add remaining seasonings except cheese and mix well. Add lettuce and toss well. Add croutons, and sprinkle with Parmesan cheese.

SERVES 4

• INSALATA CAPRESE* •

1 head romaine lettuce
1 sliced sweet onion
1 sliced ripe tomato

6 slices fresh mozzarella cheese
6 fresh basil leaves
Salt and finely ground black pepper to taste
Extra-virgin olive oil

Arrange onion on a bed of romaine. Top with a layer of sliced tomatoes, then a slice of mozzarella. Top with a fresh basil leaf. Salt and pepper to taste. Drizzle with olive oil.

SERVES 6

• CHICKPEA SALAD OR SANDWICH •

1 can chick peas or garbanzo beans
1 medium onion, finely chopped
1 red pepper, seeded and chopped
Juice of 1 lemon
1 tablespoon olive oil (if desired)
2 tablespoons Vegenaise (Follow Your Heart)
1 teaspoon cider vinegar
Fresh chopped parsley
BeauMonde seasoning to taste
Salt and pepper to taste

Drain liquid from chick peas and rinse. In a bowl, mash beans into a paste with a fork then add remaining ingredients.

Use as sandwich filling with lettuce and tomato on seven-grain bread or whole-wheat pita or on a bed of salad greens with chopped tomato and cucumber.

MAKES ABOUT 2½ CUPS OR 5 SANDWICHES

• LEMON VINAIGRETTE* •

1 cup canola oil
¼ cup fresh lemon juice
¼ cup white wine vinegar
1 clove garlic, pressed or minced
1 tablespoon finely chopped fresh chives
Salt and freshly ground pepper to taste

Put all ingredients in a jar. Cover and shake until emulsified. Keep in refrigerator.

MAKES ABOUT 1½ CUPS

• ASIAN DRESSING* •

1 cup rice vinegar
2 tablespoons light soy sauce
1 tablespoon grated fresh ginger
1½ tablespoons sesame oil
1 tablespoon sugar

Combine all ingredients in a small bowl and whisk vigorously until well blended.

MAKES ABOUT 1 CUP

• ASIAN SLAW •

1 small head red cabbage, sliced or shredded
1 small head green cabbage, sliced or shredded
2 large carrots, peeled and grated

½ cup chopped scallions

¼ cup toasted sesame seeds

DRESSING

1 cup rice vinegar

¼ teaspoon sesame oil

1 tablespoon ponzu sauce (Eden)

2 tablespoons light brown sugar

Remove and discard the cabbages' outer leaves. Shred or thinly slice and place in large bowl. Add carrots, scallions, sesame seeds, and dressing. Toss well and adjust seasonings. Allow to chill in the refrigerator.

SERVES 6

• OPEN-FACE BROILED FRESH TOMATO • AND CHEESE SANDWICH

2 tablespoons Vegenaise

½ tablespoon chipotle salsa (Frontera)

2 slices seven-grain bread

4 large slices fresh tomatoes

4 slices Pepper Jack soy cheese

Mix Vegenaise and salsa together and spread on bread. Place 2 tomato slices on top and add the cheese. Place in broiler or toaster oven until cheese is melted.

SERVES 2

• DAPHNE'S BAKED TOFU SANDWICH •

2 pounds firm tofu, rinsed and drained
2 tablespoons fresh gingerroot juice
¼ cup water
½ cup ponzu sauce
¼ cup rice vinegar
½ cup chopped scallions
2 tablespoons kudzu or cornstarch dissolved in
⅓ cup cold water

Preheat oven to 350 degrees F. Slice tofu blocks into 8 slices each. Place pieces in a lightly oiled 9 × 12-inch baking dish. Grate and squeeze ginger into a sauce pan with ponzu sauce, water, vinegar, and scallions. Bring mixture to a boil, add dissolved kudzu or cornstarch and stir until it begins to thicken. Pour mixture over tofu and bake for 35 minutes. May be served hot or cold in sandwiches.

For sandwiches, spread seven-grain bread (or your choice) with Vegenaise. Layer on large sliced tomatoes, lettuce, and baked tofu.

SERVES 4 TO 6

• VEGETARIAN CHEESE STEAK •
SANDWICHES

6 ounces seitan
1 medium sweet onion, chopped
1 clove garlic, minced
2 tablespoons olive oil
1 tablespoon Worcestershire sauce

Salt and pepper to taste
3 to 4 whole wheat French rolls
Dairy-free provolone cheese

Sauté onion and garlic in olive oil. Add sliced seitan and Worcestershire sauce to onions. Salt and pepper to taste. Split rolls; fill with seitan mixture and top with cheese. Place under broiler until cheese is melted.

SERVES 3 TO 4

• REFRIED BEAN ROLL-UPS •

1 can vegetarian refried beans
1 package taco mix
1 tomato, chopped
½ cup salad olives, chopped
1 cup shredded lettuce
4 corn tortillas
½ cup shredded soy cheese
Salsa (page 125)

Heat refried beans in a saucepan, add taco mix. Combine tomato, olives, and lettuce. Heat tortillas in foil or in clay tortilla pot in the oven. Lay flat and spread a layer of refried beans on top. Add vegetable mixture on half of the tortilla. Sprinkle with cheese and roll up. Serve with salsa.

SERVES 4

• MARGAPITA PIZZAS •

4 whole wheat pitas split open
1 cup tomato sauce, jar or homemade
Red pepper and salt to taste
8 slices fresh mozzarella cheese
12 fresh basil leaves

Cover each pita with tomato sauce. Season with pepper and salt. Top each with 2 mozzarella slices. Broil until cheese melts. Garnish with 3 basil leaves

SERVES 4

• MISO SOUP •

4 cups dashi (page 137)
¼ cup mellow white miso (may use a variety of
    miso)
¼ pound silken tofu diced into small cubes
2 teaspoons wakame flakes
2 scallions, chopped fine

Bring dashi to boil. Remove from heat. Pour ½ cup dashi into small bowl. Add miso and mix thoroughly. Add to saucepan with tofu and wakame. Do not boil. Ladle into bowls and sprinkle with chopped scallions.

SERVES 4

NOTE: For vegetarian miso soup make shiitake mushroom stock and use in place of dashi.

DASHI

1 ounce dried konbu (seaweed)

1 cup bonito flakes

6 cups water

Place seaweed in a saucepan with 6 cups water. Bring to boil and then simmer for 5 to 10 minutes. Remove seaweed and discard. Add bonito flakes to the broth plus 1 cup cold water. Bring to a boil and then simmer for 5 minutes. Remove from heat while bonito flakes settle to the bottom. Strain stock and discard bonito flakes.

MAKES ABOUT 6 CUPS

• UNCREAM OF CARROT AND GINGER SOUP •

1 large onion, chopped

1 tablespoon grated fresh ginger or finely chopped
    gingerroot, or to taste

1 tablespoon organic cold-pressed canola oil

3 cups organic carrots, peeled and diced

1 teaspoon mild curry powder, or to taste

1 medium potato, peeled and diced

6 cups water or vegetable stock

1 cup orange juice

Salt and pepper to taste

Chopped cilantro for garnish

Sauté onion and ginger in oil until translucent, about 5 minutes. Add carrots and curry powder and continue to sauté for 5 minutes. Add potato and water, bring to a boil, reduce heat, cover and simmer for about 30 minutes until carrots soften. Then stir in juice and puree in blender until smooth. If too thick, add more water or stock. Adjust seasoning. Garnish with cilantro.

SERVES 6 TO 8

• GOOD FRIDAY SOUP •

2 small zucchini, chopped

1 large potato

1 large onion, chopped

2 medium carrots, chopped

3 tablespoons chopped parsley

6 cups water or vegetable stock

2 tablespoons vegetarian chicken flavored broth
   powder, if desired

Salt and pepper to taste

Place all ingredients in a soup pot and simmer for about 45 minutes until vegetables are tender.

SERVES 4

• PASTA AND BEAN SOUP •

1 medium onion, chopped

3 tablespoons extra-virgin olive oil

5 garlic cloves, minced or crushed

3 cups chopped fresh tomatoes or 1 (28-ounce) can
   whole peeled Italian tomatoes (preferably San
   Marzano)

8 fresh basil leaves, chopped, plus whole leaves for
   garnish

6 cups water

6 ounces pasta—broken spaghetti, elbows, or tubetti

Red pepper flakes

Salt and pepper to taste

Freshly grated Parmesan cheese

Sauté onion in olive oil. When onion is golden and translucent, add garlic. Sauté for several minutes. Add tomatoes and basil. Simmer on low for 10 minutes. Add water and beans. Cook for 10 minutes. Add pasta, red pepper flakes, salt, and pepper and simmer until pasta is cooked al dente. Serve in shallow bowls, drizzle with a little extra-virgin olive oil, sprinkle with a little Parmesan cheese, and garnish with a fresh basil leaf.

SERVES 4

• ZOE'S SPLIT PEA SOUP •

8 cups water
2 cups split peas, rinsed and picked over
4 slices soy Canadian bacon, diced (Yves)
1 medium chopped onion
1 diced carrot
1 chopped potato
1 chopped celery stalk
2 chopped or pressed garlic cloves
1 tablespoon olive oil
Salt and pepper to taste

Combine all ingredients in soup pot, bring to a boil, reduce heat, and simmer gently for about 1 hour. Add more water if necessary, depending on desired thickness of soup.

SERVES 6

• MUSHROOM BARLEY AND KALE SOUP •

1 medium onion, chopped

2 celery stalks, chopped

2 cloves garlic, minced

3 cups cleaned, sliced button or shiitake mushrooms

2 tablespoons extra-virgin olive oil

1 cup barley

6 cups water

4 tablespoons vegetarian chicken broth powder

½ teaspoon thyme

½ teaspoon marjoram

Salt and pepper to taste

1 bunch kale, washed, stemmed, and chopped

Sauté onion, celery, garlic, and mushrooms in olive oil for 5 minutes. Add barley and sauté 5 minutes more. Add water and seasonings. Bring to boil. Lower heat and simmer for 45 minutes. Add kale. Simmer 15 minutes longer.

SERVES 4

• SEAFOOD CORN CHOWDER •

1 sweet onion, chopped

1 potato, diced

3 stalks celery, chopped

2 tablespoons olive oil

4 cups water

4 tablespoons vegetarian chicken broth powder

1 cup corn kernels

12 littleneck clams, washed

15 medium shrimp, cleaned

12 sea scallops

⅓ cup chopped fresh cilantro plus more for garnish

Salt and pepper to taste

Sauté onion, potato, and celery in olive oil until onion turns translucent. Add water, vegetarian chicken broth powder, and corn. Simmer for 15 minutes. Add clams, shrimp, scallops, and cilantro. Bring to boil, reduce heat and simmer until seafood is done and clams have fully opened. Add salt and pepper to taste. Sprinkle with cilantro.

SERVES 4

• OAT BRAN BANANA NUT MUFFINS •

¼ cup raisins

2 cups oat bran hot cereal uncooked

1 tablespoon baking powder

¼ cup chopped walnuts

1 teaspoon ground cinnamon

¼ teaspoon ground allspice

½ cup molasses

2 ripe bananas, mashed

2 egg whites, slightly beaten

1¼ cups skim milk (or vanilla rice or soy milk)

2 tablespoons cold-pressed organic canola oil

½ cup shredded carrot

Cover raisins with boiling water. Let stand for 5 minutes, drain, and set aside.

In a large mixing bowl stir together oat bran, baking powder, nuts, cinnamon, allspice, and molasses. In a medium bowl combine mashed bananas, egg whites, milk, and canola oil. Add all at once to the bran mixture until just moistened. The batter should be lumpy. Fold in raisins and carrot.

Fill paper baking cups two-thirds full. Bake at 400 degrees F for 18 to 20 minutes or until golden. Serve warm.

MAKES 6 MUFFINS

• LESS THE YOLK OMELET •

1 stalk celery, finely chopped
1 red or green bell pepper, finely chopped
1 sweet onion, finely chopped
2 slices Pepper Jack soy cheese
1 tablespoon canola oil
3 egg whites
Salt and freshly ground black pepper

Sauté vegetables in oil in a nonstick pan until onion is transparent. Remove from pan and set aside. Beat egg whites slightly. Heat same pan with canola oil on medium heat. Add egg whites. Cook until eggs begin to set. Add vegetables and cheese to one side and fold in half. Put lid over pan and cook until cheese melts. Salt and pepper to taste.

VARIATION: *One to Three Omelet* Follow above recipe, but add 1 yolk to 3 egg whites.

SERVES 1

• ROSEMARY BREAKFAST POTATOES •

4 to 5 medium-size potatoes, cut into bite-size
    pieces
4 tablespoons olive oil
Fresh or dried rosemary leaves
Salt and pepper to taste

Lightly oil a cookie sheet. Toss potatoes lightly in olive oil. Sprinkle with dried or fresh rosemary, salt, and pepper. Bake at 350 degrees F for 30 minutes or until nicely browned.

SERVES 2 TO 4

• TOFU SCRAMBLE* •

1 small sweet onion, chopped
1 clove garlic, minced
½ green bell pepper, chopped
½ red bell pepper, chopped
2 tablespoons extra-virgin olive oil or canola oil
2 pounds tofu, crumbled
1 teaspoon turmeric
2 tablespoons chopped fresh parsley or fresh cilantro
Salt and pepper to taste

Sauté onion, garlic, and green and red peppers in oil until softened. Drain tofu; add to vegetables and break it up with a fork to desired consistency. Add turmeric, parsley, and salt and pepper to taste.

SERVES 4

• PORTUGUESE BAKED COD WITH RICE •

2 tablespoons olive oil

6 tomatoes, chopped

2 garlic cloves, pressed or minced

1 small onion, finely chopped

½ cup chopped black olives

2 tablespoons chopped cilantro plus a few sprigs for
    garnish

3 pounds cod fish

½ cup cooked brown rice

Salt and pepper to taste

1 cup dry white wine

Preheat oven to 350 degrees F.

Pour the oil into a shallow baking dish. Scatter half the tomatoes, garlic, onion, black olives, and cilantro in the dish. Put the fish and rice on top, season with salt and pepper and cover with the rest of the tomatoes, garlic, onion, black olives, and cilantro. Pour the wine on top. Bake for 35 to 45 minutes, basting often. Place on a warm serving plate. If necessary boil drippings to thicken and pour over fish. Garnish with cilantro sprigs.

SERVES 6

• HORIZONS CAFÉ •
FAT-FREE SEITAN STEAK MARSALA
Through the kindness of Chef Richard Landau

½ inch dry Marsala wine on the bottom of a large
    skillet or wok

½ cup vegetable broth

Garlic, to taste

Fresh herbs (rosemary, thyme, or basil)

Chopped onions or leeks

3 ounces seitan, quickly rinsed with cold water

Mushrooms

1 teaspoon arrowroot or cornstarch to thicken

Salt and pepper to taste

Preheat skillet with wine and broth to a simmer over medium heat. Add garlic, herbs, and onions. Slowly add seitan. Add mushrooms and simmer for 7 minutes or until mushrooms are tender. Season with salt and pepper.

In a separate dish, mix arrowroot with water (until there are no lumps). Add arrowroot mixture to the pan and stir. Allow to thicken, stirring occasionally, approximately 3 to 4 minutes. Serve with brown rice and steamed vegetables.

SERVES 1

• HORIZONS CAFÉ •
FAT-FREE SEITAN POT ROAST
Through the kindness of Chef Richard Landau

3 ounces seitan, quickly rinsed with cold water

Baby red potatoes (small)

Baby carrots

Whole mushrooms

Sliced wild mushrooms (shiitake or portobello)

Garlic, to taste

½ cup vegetable broth

¼ cup dry white wine

Fresh thyme and rosemary

Salt and pepper to taste

Preheat oven to 450 degrees F. Place all ingredients together in a large roast-
ing pan. Cover with foil and bake for 15 minutes or until the potatoes are
tender.

SERVES 1

• PORTLAND COUNTRY CLUB'S •
SAKÉ-GLAZED SEA BASS

> 8 ounces sea bass
> Ginger slices
> 1 cup sake
> ½ cup sugar
> ¼ cup juice from pickled ginger
> 1 tablespoon pickled ginger

Rinse and pat dry sea bass. Poke holes in the skin side with a knife. Place
a slice of ginger in each hole. Salt and pepper all sides and pan-sear in an
ovenproof sauté pan.

In a saucepan combine saké, sugar, juice from pickled ginger, and pickled
ginger. Simmer and reduce by half. Let cool.

Drizzle the saké mixture over the sea bass and place in a 350-degree F
oven for 10 to 15 minutes.

SERVES 1 OR 2

• SEARED TUNA •

> 2 pounds fresh tuna
> ⅓ cup olive oil
> ½ cup soy sauce

¼ cup ponzu sauce (Eden)

1 teaspoon honey

½ teaspoon grated fresh ginger

2 cloves garlic

4 scallions, chopped

Cracked pepper to taste

Cut tuna into four pieces. Combine remaining ingredients in a large bowl, and marinate tuna in the liquid for 2 hours. Heat skillet and cook tuna for 2 minutes on each side (longer if you desire).

SERVES 4

• FESTIVE SALMON ROLL* •

Large salmon fillet

2 cups cooked spinach

½ cup feta cheese

¼ cup pine nuts

Salt and freshly ground pepper

2 tablespoons extra-virgin olive oil

2 garlic cloves, minced or pressed

Remove the skin from a large salmon fillet. Cover the fillet with spinach, feta cheese, and pine nuts. Salt and pepper to taste. Place in baking dish that has been lightly oiled. Mix olive oil and garlic. Spoon mixture over salmon. Roll fillet from one end to the other making a log. Tie with string in 3 or 4 places. Bake at 375 degrees F for 20 to 30 minutes, depending on desired degree of doneness. Slice from roll, removing string.

SERVES 4 TO 6, DEPENDING ON SIZE OF FILLET

• VEGETARIAN SAUSAGE AND •
ZUCCHINI SAUTÉ

1 sweet onion, chopped
2 tablespoons olive oil or canola oil
4 medium zucchinis, chopped
2 vegetarian sausages
2 tomatoes, chopped
Salt and pepper to taste
Red (cayenne) pepper (optional)

Sauté onion in oil until semisoft. Add zucchini and sausage and sauté for 5 to 7 minutes. Add tomatoes. Add salt and pepper and a dash of red pepper, to taste.

SERVES 4

• JERRY'S FAVORITE PASTA •
(SPINACH AND ANGEL HAIR)

2 tablespoons olive oil
2 cloves garlic, pressed or minced
8 cups fresh spinach, or 3 packages frozen
1 pound angel hair pasta (whole wheat if possible)
1 cup water
2 tablespoons vegetarian chicken broth powder
Salt and pepper to taste

Heat a pot of water for pasta. In a sauté pan, heat olive oil and add garlic. When soft but not browned, add spinach and continue to sauté. Put pasta in boiling water and cook following directions on package. Add water and broth powder to spinach. Season with salt and pepper. Simmer for 5 minutes. Serve over pasta.

SERVES 4

• MEATLESS BALLS •

1 package Gimme Lean (beef), crumbled
1 medium onion, finely diced
1 clove garlic, pressed or minced
⅓ cup Italian bread crumbs
½ teaspoon dried oregano
1 egg white
Salt and pepper to taste
3 tablespoons olive oil

Place the Gimme Lean in a large bowl. Add all ingredients except the olive oil and mix together. Roll into 18 balls and brown in olive oil.

MAKES 18 "MEAT" BALLS

• CHARLIE'S TOMATO SAUCE* •

¼ cup extra-virgin olive oil
6 cloves garlic, finely chopped
1 medium onion, finely chopped
1 (64-ounce) can whole peeled Italian tomatoes
2 (28-ounce) cans crushed tomatoes
1 teaspoon oregano
1 teaspoon fennel powder
¼ teaspoon sugar
4 fresh basil leaves, chopped
1 teaspoon fresh chopped parsley
Red pepper flakes, if desired
Salt and pepper to taste
Parmesan cheese, if desired

Heat the olive oil in a large saucepan. Sauté garlic and onions until translucent. Add the remaining ingredients except the pasta and Parmesan. Cook for 1 hour. Purée with hand blender. Serve over pasta and sprinkle with Parmesan cheese if desired.

MAKES ABOUT 15 CUPS

• FRESH TOMATO SAUCE •

4 large ripe tomatoes
¾ cup fresh basil leaves, shredded
2 cloves garlic, minced
½ cup extra-virgin olive oil
Salt and freshly ground pepper to taste

Chop tomatoes. Place in a mixing bowl with basil, garlic, and oil. Salt and pepper to taste. Allow flavors to marry for 1 hour. Serve over pasta.

SERVES 4

• CHRISTOPHER'S MARINADE •

½ cup ponzu sauce (Eden) or low-sodium soy sauce
  (Kikkoman)
½ cup rice vinegar
1 tablespoon light brown sugar
1 teaspoon dark roasted sesame oil
1 teaspoon lemon or lime juice
2 garlic cloves, minced or pressed
1 tablespoon gingerroot juice (grated and squeezed)

Combine all ingredients. Use as a marinade.

MAKES ABOUT 1 CUP

• DON'T WORRY CURRY •

1 cup brown lentils, sorted and washed
1 cup brown rice, rinsed
4 cups water
4 tablespoons vegetarian chicken broth powder
4 thin slices fresh ginger
3 stalks celery, finely chopped
3 garlic cloves, finely chopped
1 red bell pepper, chopped
1 to 2 tablespoons curry powder, mild or hot
Salt and pepper to taste

Place all ingredients in electric rice cooker or in pot on stove. Bring to a full boil, then turn to low and simmer for 1 hour or until liquid is absorbed.

SERVES 4 TO 6

• SPANISH RICE •

1 onion, chopped

1 green bell pepper, cored, seeded, and chopped

4 tablespoons extra-virgin olive oil

1 cup basmati rice

1 tablespoon spicy mustard

1 (8-ounce) can tomato sauce

2¾ cups water

Salt and freshly ground pepper to taste

½ package taco seasoning

Cook onions and green pepper in oil. Add rice and stir. Add mustard and stir. Add tomato sauce, 2 cups water, and some salt. Bring this mixture to a boil and simmer, covered, for 30 minutes. Add more water if needed. Remove from heat when liquid is absorbed.

Sprinkle with taco seasoning and add the ¾ cup water. Cook until water is absorbed. Add mixture to rice. Mix thoroughly, reheat, and serve.

SERVES 6

• CHRISTOPHER'S RICE •

1 tablespoon cold-pressed organic canola oil

2 tablespoons minced or pressed garlic

1 teaspoon Asian chili paste (available in Asian stores)

1 teaspoon light brown sugar

2 tablespoons ponzu sauce (Eden)

1 tablespoon Asian fish sauce (available in Asian
   stores)

6 cups cooked jasmine rice

1 cup fresh Thai basil leaves (available in Asian stores)

Heat oil in a wok or large saucepan. Sauté garlic until fragrant but not brown. Add chili paste, sugar, ponzu sauce, and fish sauce and stir well to combine ingredients. Add rice and basil. Stir-fry for 5 minutes until thoroughly heated.

SERVES 4

• BROCCOLI BAOBABS* •

2 cloves garlic, chopped

⅓ cup olive oil

Red pepper flakes

1 large head broccoli

½ fresh lemon

Salt, black pepper

Sauté garlic in olive oil until golden (not browned). Add red pepper flakes to taste (start with a pinch). Steam broccoli until light green and tender. Drizzle olive oil mixture over broccoli. Finish with squeeze of lemon and salt and pepper to taste.

SERVES 4

• STUFFED ACORN SQUASH •

2 acorn squash, halved and seeded
1 tablespoon organic cold-pressed canola oil
1 package Gimme Lean (sausage flavor)
1 medium onion, finely chopped
2 celery stalks, finely chopped
Salt and pepper to taste
2 tablespoons finely chopped parsley
4 tablespoons grated Parmesan cheese or 4 slices
    pepper jack soy cheese

Place squash upside down in baking pan with a half inch of water in bottom of pan. Cover with foil. Bake in 375 degrees F oven for 30 minutes.

Meanwhile, prepare the stuffing. Heat oil in a large saucepan. Sauté the Gimme Lean until browned. Add onions and celery and sauté for 5 minutes, until softened. Season with salt and pepper and stir in parsley.

When squash are done, remove from pan. Turn squash right side up and fill with stuffing. Top each half with 1 tablespoon Parmesan cheese or 1 slice of soy cheese. Bake for 30 minutes and serve.

SERVES 4

• FRENCH UNFRIES •

4 russet potatoes, scrubbed
Canola oil in a pump spray
Salt to taste

Preheat oven to 375 degrees F.

Cut the scrubbed, unpeeled potatoes into french-fry size. Spray a large baking sheet with canola oil in a pump spray. Arrange potatoes without overlapping them. Spray with oil and bake for 1 hour and 20 minutes. Turn after 30 minutes and then frequently until crisp and brown. Add salt as desired.

SERVES 4

• CUCUMBER YOGURT RAITA •

1 cup plain low-fat or nonfat yogurt
1 cucumber, peeled, seeded, and finely chopped
2 cloves garlic, pressed
Salt and white pepper to taste

Combine all ingredients. If possible refrigerate for several hours before serving.

SERVES 2

• SPICY ASIAN SAUCE •

2½ cups water
2 tablespoons vegetarian broth powder
2 tablespoons ponzu sauce (Eden)
2 tablespoons black bean garlic paste
½ teaspoon freshly ground black pepper
⅓ cup cornstarch
¾ cup water
2 teaspoons toasted sesame oil
½ cup chopped cilantro

In a saucepan combine water, vegetarian broth powder, ponzu sauce, black-bean paste, and pepper. Bring to a boil, reduce heat, and simmer on low for 5 minutes.

Mix cornstarch and water in a small bowl and stir until smooth. Stir into mixture and simmer until sauce thickens. Stir occasionally. Remove from heat. Add sesame oil and cilantro. Pour over seafood and noodles.

MAKES ABOUT 4 CUPS

• STEWED PRUNES •

1 English Breakfast tea bag
9 prunes, pitted or not
2 lemon slices
1 cup water
¼ teaspoon sugar

Make the tea in a saucepan. Add remaining ingredients. Bring to boil and simmer for about 30 minutes

SERVES 3

• SOY FLAX SHAKE •

1 cup vanilla soy milk
2 tablespoons ground flax seeds
½ banana, or any desired fruit (pears, strawberries,
    kiwis, etc.)

Place all ingredients in blender and blend until smooth.

MAKES 1 SHAKE

• MAGIC DRINK •

1½ cups juice—orange, grapefruit, natural cranberry,
   apple, pineapple, etc.
½ banana
¼ teaspoon vitamin C crystals
1 tablespoon flaxseed oil
1 to 3 teaspoons psyllium husks
1 scoop soy protein powder
1 teaspoon nutritional yeast

OPTIONAL
Kiwis
Strawberries
Peaches
1 tablespoon Green Magma Plus

Combine ingredients in blender and blend until smooth.

MAKES 1 SHAKE

• COOL GREEN MAGIC DRINK •

2 cups orange juice

2 kiwis

½ banana

6 strawberries (optional)

1 teaspoon psyllium seed husks

1 tablespoon Veggie Magma

1 tablespoon Magma Plus

1 tablespoon soy protein

1 tablespoon multivitamins and mineral powder

1 tablespoon flaxseed oil

½ teaspoon vitamin C crystals

Put all ingredients in a blender and add 1 cup ice. Blend well.

SERVES 3

• FRUIT JUICE SODAS •

Add fruit juice—cranberry juice, lime, orange, grapefruit, etc.—to sparkling water. Garnish with a piece of the fruit. (Use a natural sweetner, Stevia, if more sweetness is desired.)

7

Exercise and Massage

EXERCISE

Integrative medicine has finally come to realize the importance of exercise to health, and particularly to cardiac health. Our advice to cardiac patients and postoperative patients used to be to lie still "until you have a chance to get better." Now we have them up and walking on the day after the operation. Our whole country has become exercise conscious, and the proliferation of health clubs, in-home machines such as Nordic Tracks and stairmasters, and personal trainers testifies to the fact that at least one large segment of the population is aware of the benefits of exercise. (A different segment is content—often belligerently so—to remain couch potatoes.)

Regular exercise increases lean muscle mass and strength, raises the basal metabolic rate, maintains weight loss, decreases resting heart rate and blood pressure, lowers LDL and elevates HDL, increases the flow of oxygen and blood to muscles and coronary arteries, and in general optimizes heart function. Sometimes I feel like an old New England preacher when I say these things, but in my opinion every healthy person who does not exercise regularly is committing a sin against his or her body. (There are, however, factors to be aware of if you're a cardiac patient. Extreme exercise will increase oxidative stress and reduce levels of antioxidants and CoQ_{10} in the body. And unlike muscle tone and physical fitness, cardiovascular tone requires only about half an hour of daily walking to achieve good results.)

My recommendations:

- *Walk* for thirty minutes a day, keeping the arms moving and going along at a pace of 3.5 to 4 miles per hour. This is just as beneficial to your lymphatic health as running, and the advantage to walking is that it causes less stress to the joints. For many, especially the elderly or people suffering from arthritis, running or jogging can be painful. For some, even walking may be difficult, but if you can do it without pain, it should be your first option.
- *Swim* whenever you can. This form of exercise is particularly beneficial to the elderly since it puts least strain on the joints. Half an hour's swim, without pushing yourself, is an ideal conditioner.
- *Run* or *jog* if you're so inclined, or play basketball, tennis, soccer, even golf. Anything that keeps you moving.
- *Make love.* Yes, sex is good exercise, and good for the lymphatics, but those past a certain age need other forms of exercise to supplement it.
- *Jump* on a trampoline or "rebounder." This is a form of exercise particularly suited to the lymphatic system, and it has the advantage that you can do it at home or in the office. (I keep a trampoline in my own office and use it daily.) I recommend beginning with 100 jumping jacks daily (about five minutes). Beginning

with arms at your sides and legs together, jump up and come down with legs spread and arms over your head. Then jump up and return to your original position. Over several weeks you might want to bring the number of jumps to 500, but don't try them at all if you have poor balance or are in any way disabled. You can still get benefit from a trampoline by sitting on it and bouncing up and down.

- *Meditate.* A good way to combine meditation with exercise is to lie on the floor, tensing and then relaxing first your toes, then your legs, then your pelvis, abdomen, chest, upper arms, lower arms, hands, neck, head, face, and scalp. When you're fully relaxed, rid your mind of thoughts, letting whatever happens happen.

No matter what exercise you choose, the important thing is to do it regularly and habitually. Studies in the United States and Japan showed a twofold decrease in mortality and complications of coronary artery disease in patients who walked regularly compared with those who did not. No matter what exercise you prefer, the key is consistency.

Again, though, a caveat. If you haven't been exercising and are now inspired to do so, get a stress test (from your doctor) to rule out the possibility of silent coronary artery disease.

Exercise and the Lymphatics

Exercise is a powerful conditioner of the lymphatic system. We've already seen the vital part the lymphatics play in arteriosclerosis and other coronary diseases and the importance of clearing lipoproteins and toxic substances from the arterial wall. Lymphatic fluid, which has a larger volume than blood, circulates throughout the body once every day, and 50 percent of the body's lipoproteins pass through the lymphatic system daily. Exercise can increase lymphatic flow threefold (or more with extreme exercise), thus increasing the clearance of lipoproteins, peptides, and glycoproteins from the arterial wall. It's easy math to see that by increasing your exercise, you can increase the circulation of HDL in the bloodstream, thus mobilizing more cholesterol from the arterial wall.

One of the side effects of exercise is, of course, perspiration. As it is secreted, sweat takes with it some of the metabolites that would otherwise stay in our tissue. A sauna taken after exercise (or even without exercise) aids the process.

All exercise is good for the lymphatics; a brisk 2-mile walk each day will keep the circulation flowing. But in addition to the most commonly practiced forms of exercise, other forms, mostly derived from the East, are becoming more and more popular here.

YOGA Originating in India, yoga is actually more a spiritual practice than a physical exercise, though we in the West tend to use it to improve posture and breathing. The word means "yoking together in union," and the practice is believed to be the link between body and soul, melding the two facets of the human being. Yoga exercises have been shown to improve blood pressure, hypertension, heart rate, breathing, and mental attitude. Yoga can contribute to the reduction of heart disease by reducing stress, anxiety, and hypertension while improving muscular strength and self-confidence. In one study, after three months of practicing yoga and receiving biofeedback, 25 percent of the patients were able to discontinue their antihypertensive drugs and another 35 percent were able to decrease the dosage by up to 60 percent. Yoga is particularly valuable for older people because of the minimal impact imposed on the skeleton. Like other forms of exercise, it increases lymphatic flow.

I'll have more to say about yoga—and will present several yoga exercises—in the next chapter.

TAI CHI A gentle form of martial art in the Chinese tradition, tai chi is a series of motions and postures that promotes harmony of the mind and body through relaxed breathing and mental focus. Psychological, respiratory, and cardiovascular improvement, as well as improved balance, have been documented in several studies. Improved endurance and oxygen consumption, often concomitant with moderate exercise, have also been documented. Tai chi is widely used in the Orient for cardiovascular fitness and is an especially good exercise for elderly people because of its low impact on the skeleton.

CHI GONG Chi gong is similar to tai chi, with a greater focus on realigning the body's energy forces. It also involves a series of postures and movements that are reported to improve the body's energy. Chi gong has been shown to have a beneficial effect on the immune system, on the gastrointestinal tract, and on chronic degenerative diseases such as hypertension, arthritis, and coronary heart disease.

•　•　•

In sum, when it comes specifically to lymphatic health, most forms of exercise are beneficial, which is why I advocate a daily regimen in my overall program. Ideally, I recommend, daily:

- A 2-mile walk at 3.5 to 4 miles per hour (thirty minutes)
- 100 jumping jacks on a trampoline (five minutes)
- Basic yoga postures (twenty minutes)
- Meditation (five minutes minimum)

The important thing to remember is that exercise is as important as diet, breathing, and spirituality in the balance of factors that promote good health. Exercise as it suits you. But *exercise.*

MASSAGE

What does an athlete get before taking to the field or the pool? A massage. And what after? Again, a massage. The first massage is to prevent injuries, the second to relax muscles and bones made tense by the exercise—to restore the body's equilibrium.

Pregnant women benefit from massage; it soothes strained muscles and relaxes them before they give birth. Little babies love to be massaged—it encourages bonding with the parent, reduces crying and colic, and lulls them to sleep. The elderly, too, enjoy massage, particularly of the back and neck muscles and the feet.

Today massage has become a common therapy not only for the above groups but for everybody. For many years Americans tended to overlook it, relying instead on drugs and machines to ease their pains and fears, but now it has become an accepted and highly recommended medical practice. I can think of no therapy more pleasurable, no preventive more relaxing, no regimen more passionately anticipated.

Massage will be of enormous value to anyone suffering from stress or fatigue (probably 99 percent of the population). A recent study at the University of Miami Medical School showed that workers who underwent twenty-minute therapeutic massages twice a week reported less tiredness and more clearheadedness. Indeed, some employers hire freelance massage therapists for those who request them, often paying all—more usually half—of the therapist's bill.

Massage has more direct medical benefits as well. It reduces congestion and improves circulation; it increases the flow of oxygen and micronutrients to muscles, joints, and the brain; it aids elimination of metabolic waste; it may cure insomnia; and it reduces pain. (What do you do when you bang your leg against a table? You rub it.)

Massage has been used as a therapeutic tool as far back as the ancient Chinese, Japanese, Egyptians, Greeks, and Romans. It works because the soft tissues—muscles, ligaments, tendons, and fascia—respond to touch, and most pain is felt most severely in those tissues. When applied to trigger points—those places in the muscles that evoke pain in various parts of the body—massage can reduce tightness and pain. Most headaches originate in the muscles of the neck. Abdominal and pelvic pain is usually caused by trigger points in the muscles of those regions. Lower back pain and sciatica are far more likely to come from the muscles than the vertebrae. Bad posture can misalign the muscles and bones and be a cause of constant pain. Massage, more than drugs and more than corrective surgery, can relieve pain, and I'm talking about emotional and well as physical pain. In Germany, massage is prescribed by doctors and paid for by insurance.

Some medical conditions, including cancer, open wounds, acute back pain, and bacterial or viral diseases, cannot be helped by massage. But for everything else, including the simple rigors of daily existence, massage is a lifesaver. And when massage is administered by a loving partner, a oneness is felt that can be of enormous psychological benefit to both parties. Mind-body therapists such as Ilana Rubenfeld have proved the psychological benefits of touch. It need not be sexual touch; gentle massage can communicate a profound message of love.

Massage and the Lymphatics

Because lymph flows it is open to massage, and in fact there is a special technique, pioneered by the Danish therapists Emil and Estrid Vodder in the 1930s, that is particularly used to stimulate circulation of the lymph. Called Manual Lymphatic Drainage (MLD), it is a way of gently palpating and moving the skin to treat the entire lymphatic system. It can be used for a variety of ailments, helping to bring down swelling and bruising, relieve sinus congestion, reduce water retention and cellulite, and ease arthritic pain. It may even strengthen the immune system.

If MLD is to work, it must be done frequently. You can do it by yourself or with a partner, alternating the roles of therapist and subject. (But treatment of serious problems such as the edemas—swellings in the limbs—associated with breast cancer, heart failure, or thrombosis, you'll need a professional masseur.)

There is a right way and a wrong way to do MLD. The following illustrations show the direction the skin should be moved on

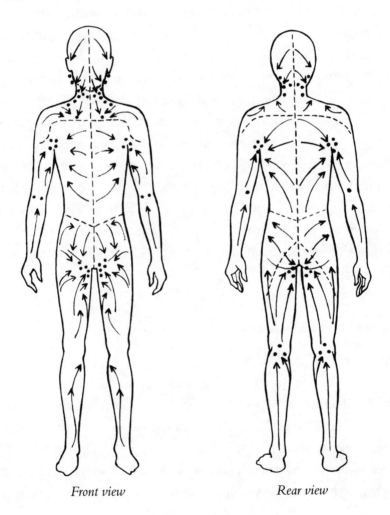

Front view   *Rear view*

the body to improve the flow of lymph toward the lymph nodes or toward the area most in need of treatment.

FACE AND NECK Here is an exercise to make your skin firmer and help eliminate puffiness. Make sure your movements are light and soft, and begin at the neck, where many of the lymph nodes are located.

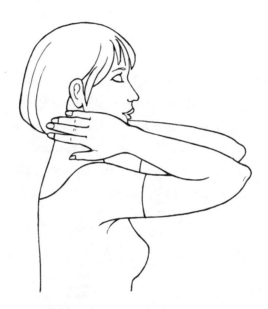

1. With your elbows raised at right angles to your body, place your hands as shown in the diagram. Use the middle part of your fingers to move the skin gently up and down in a circular motion, then release. Do this five times, then move your hands down an inch and perform the movement again, remembering to keep your fingers straight and relaxed. Then cross your arms over your chest and work the tops of your shoulders, moving the skin forward and releasing it in a circular motion. Repeat this entire exercise a minimum of three times.

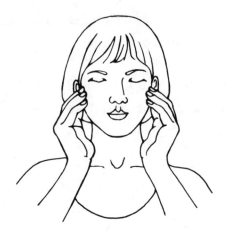

2. Make your "skin circles" on either side of your jaw, moving toward your ears. Always move the skin toward your body and let the skin naturally move your fingers back. Perform the exercise a minimum of three times, then move your fingers so they can make gentle circles on the rest of your face, employing all your fingers for the flat areas, the index and third fingers alone on the sides of your nose.

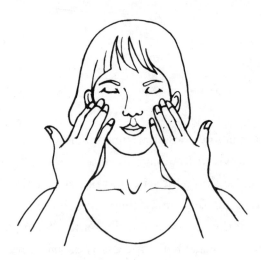

3. For puffiness around the eyes, place your hands as shown in the illustration; using just the pads of your fingers, apply light

pressure—little more than a butterfly kiss—to the area between the eyes and the cheekbone. This exercise helps with problems of discoloration as well.

You and a Partner

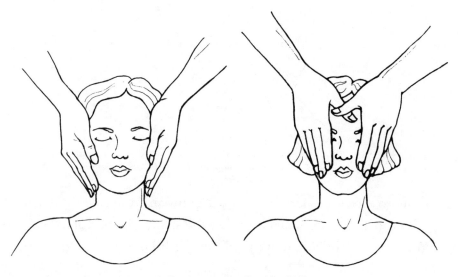

Stationary Circles (for face)

FACE

1. Sit quietly in a comfortable position. Your partner will stand over you; with her fingers placed as shown, she will gently make five "skin circles." Again, the skin will be moved toward the body, then toward the ears, and then released. Repeat a minimum of three times.

2. Your partner will place his fingers on either side of the mouth, as in the illustration, and use them to make skin circles on the remainder of your face.

BACK

1. Stand comfortably. With fingers pointed upward and thumbs at right angles on either side of the spine, your partner will use her

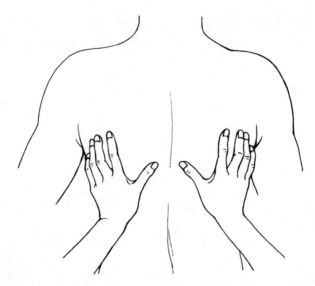

Rotary Movements (for back)

palms to move the skin gently up, then toward your sides, and then release, maintaining contact so that the skin pulls the hands back. Your partner should always work up the back toward your heart. Repeat.

2. Use the same exercise for the chest and abdomen.

LEGS

1. Sit comfortably. Have your partner make "skin circles" around the groin area, always moving the skin toward the body. Your partner will then bend your knee, placing one hand on the front of your leg, the other behind it, as shown.

2. Your partner will perform a pump action by using the front hand to softly move the skin toward the outside of your leg, then gently lift the skin upward with the palm.

3. Then, the scoop: your partner will move the skin upward with a gentle scooping motion. He will alternate pumps and scoops, continuing up to the knee. Repeat a minimum of three times.

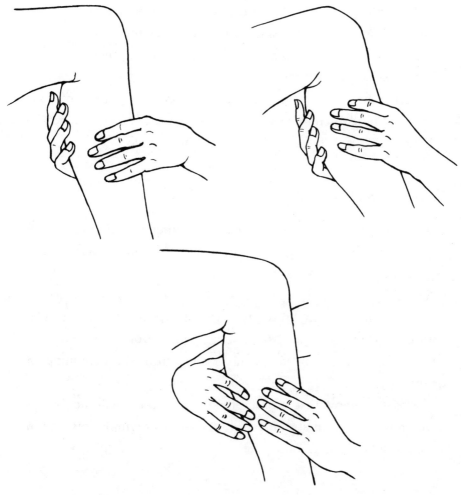

Pump and Scoop (for legs)

Note that all these exercises are used not only to benefit the skin but also for relaxation. When your partner has finished, change places so that you become the masseuse or masseur.

Simple Exercises to Alleviate Discomfort

1. For arthritic hands, softly massage between the tendons from the knuckles to the wrist.

2. For stress, have your partner give you a back massage, with particular attention to the shoulders and neck, which is where most tension is held. Knead as you would bread dough, then end with soft strokes for relaxation.

3. For headache, have your partner massage the back of your neck and head, then move to the forehead, the temples, and around the eyes. Make sure the massage is light and gentle.

Calming Strokes

Stroking is the easiest of all massage techniques, and it can be as calming and beneficial as a deep massage from a professional. While there are many kinds of stroking (including "cat," "aura," "fan," "circle," "deep," and a number of Chinese techniques), all recommend an increase in pressure as you go toward the heart. The stroking needn't be heavy or rough; a gentle stroking of one partner by another has been giving pleasure from the beginning of time.

We now know that stroking the neck of a dog will increase its lymph flow. Overall, stroking will increase your lymph flow, and in the nicest way you can imagine.

•   •   •

One of the keystones of stress management, exercise, massage, and meditation is breathing. It is so important to overall health that it is worth an entire chapter (with a little yoga—where proper breathing is vital—thrown in).

8

Breathing and Yoga

BREATHING

Proper breathing is the most important thing you can do for maintaining health. "But I breathe all the time," you might say. "It's an unconscious process. Everybody knows that the first sign of death is that breathing stops."

True enough. But if that's your attitude, you're overlooking the word *proper*. For there are different ways to breathe—indeed, a right way and a wrong way.

Breathing is the one essential and vital function over which we have most control. We can't direct how our kidneys or liver should function without great difficulty. But we have the potential to master with ease the depth and rate of breathing, which then affects our heart rate—and even our thinking. "Take a deep breath," we tell ourselves before going into a stressful situation or when we want to calm down after a trauma or strenuous exercise. It's an expression people have used for centuries, for we know that a deep

CHEST DYNAMICS IN BREATHING

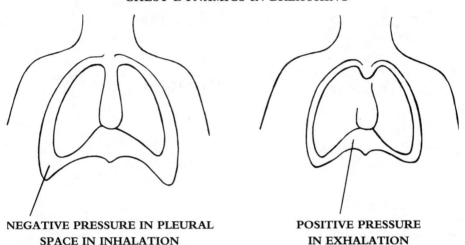

NEGATIVE PRESSURE IN PLEURAL   **POSITIVE PRESSURE**
SPACE IN INHALATION   **IN EXHALATION**

breath will ease the mind, slow down anxiety, and reduce the heart rate. Quite simply, if you master your breath, you master your health.

The Function of Breathing

Breathing's main purpose is to exchange oxygen for carbon dioxide in the lungs. The lungs act as a bellows. The muscles of the chest and diaphragm, when they are activated by breathing, expand the chest cavity, or thorax, and the lungs follow. The pressure in the space between the lung and the chest wall is dependent on whether you are inhaling or exhaling. During inhalation, the pressure is markedly negative; during exhalation, it can be positive. This sets up a pumping action, and the thoracic duct—the channel through which the lymph flows from the heart and throughout the body—can do its work.

Our lungs are connected to our nervous system by a series of nerves that monitor the level of oxygen and carbon dioxide in our body. If the oxygen level drops or the carbon dioxide level increases, this is sensed in the nervous system and the brain, which then tell the lungs to increase or deepen the breathing volume and rate and thus raise the oxygen or lower the carbon dioxide.

Breathing for normal people is driven by the level of carbon dioxide in the blood. As the carbon dioxide builds up, it sets off a response in the brain that drives a person to breathe more, thus getting rid of the carbon dioxide. In people with chronic lung disease or smokers, however, the carbon dioxide level is always high. Their breathing then is driven by the level of *oxygen* in the blood. As it goes down, the brain sends out signals for the lungs to breathe, but the accumulated carbon dioxide is not completely eliminated.

How to Breathe

If you watch young children, you'll see that they breathe from their diaphragm, the muscle that separates the upper body from the lower. Yet as we get older and are prey to anxiety, stress, or fear, our breathing shifts to the chest and becomes more rapid and more shallow. If you can consciously shift breathing back to the diaphragm, you will naturally breathe more deeply. I urge you to try it.

Here are three exercises that will help you breathe more deeply. If you're an older person, try one or two sets at first until you're comfortable, and then increase the number. Try to practice the exercises every day. They will take only a few minutes of your time, and their benefits may be immeasurable.

1. Extend your arms in front of your body, touch your palms together, and then take in a deep breath through your nose. As you do, bring your arms out to the side so that they are fully extended in a T fashion. Hold your breath for a count of four, then exhale slowly, bringing your arms back in front, palms touching. (If you've

ever watched orchestra conductors, you'll know why theirs is the longest-lived profession. They move their upper extremities in time with their breath, which helps lymphatic flow from the heart. And of course, they are focused and fixed on responding to music rather than wasting time and energy on negative thoughts and emotions.)

2. Either sitting or preferably standing or walking, inhale. Count to four. Exhale. Count to five. Repeat.

3. Take a deep breath through your mouth. Hold it as long as you can, then blow it out as much as you can. At that point, see if you can exhale just a little bit more. Usually you'll find that the extra effort helps, and the exhalation will be greater than you thought possible. On the next inhalation, do the same thing. Exhale as far as you can—and then just a little bit more. This exercise will slowly train the muscles of your chest and lungs to expand to greater volumes and will enable your body to get used to the performance of deep breathing.

Naturally, you aren't going to go through a day thinking about breathing—you'd have little time for anything else. But if you take a few minutes in the morning or before you go to bed (or both) to exercise your breathing, you'll find that soon you'll be taking deeper breaths throughout the day. Caution: Don't overdo or increase rapidly. Hyperventilation can cause dizziness or syncope (fainting).

Breathing and Toxins

One danger of deep breathing is that we inhale the noxious chemicals that are hourly pumped into our atmosphere in ever-increasing amounts. Over 500 million tons of petrochemical waste products are released into the air every year, about ten times more than at the end of World War II. Products like DDT and PCB are also harmful because when taken into our system through breathing they produce an inflammatory reaction, may have a hormonal effect, and can exacerbate asthma. And since they are oil-based, they are absorbed by the fats and lipids in our cell membranes and can thus cause a mutation of the DNA molecules or lead to cancer.

We all know by now that smoking is a leading cause of cancer and heart disease, but few understand why. First, mechanically, it destroys the *cilia*, small hairlike outgrowths of the trachea, or windpipe. The cilia gently move mucus upward so that it does not plug the air sacs where oxygen is exchanged for carbon dioxide. When the cilia are destroyed, mucus is retained in the lungs, a setup for pneumonia or obstructive lung disease. Second, smoking depletes the vitamin C in our system, setting up a susceptibility to oxidative stress. Third, smoking causes spasm of the pulmonary and arterial walls, which produces constriction and wheezing, decreased oxygen transport, and spasm of the arteries themselves, with attendant hypertension of the lungs and the body in general. Fourth, smoking causes an inflammatory reaction in the lungs and a mutation of the DNA molecule, which sets up a predisposition to cancer. And last, smoking causes spasms of the lymphatics of the lung.

So don't smoke, and if you're smoking now, stop. It's a tired command, an oft-repeated warning, but if it were up to me I'd show every preteenager slides of smokers' lungs and force them to watch, as I have, otherwise sane people die in agony because they couldn't stop smoking. Smoking *is addictive;* for most people, it is very difficult to quit. Hence the lesson for preteens. You don't have to stop what you never start.

It's more and more difficult to find clean air, but for city dwellers, I urge the use of air purifiers in the home and office, and for those of you lucky enough to live in the relatively pollution-free country, I advise long walks outdoors. Here particularly, deep breathing helps clear the toxins and metabolic wastes from everyday life that travel through the lymphatic system to be processed by the kidneys and liver. The psychological benefits are apparent as well. Inhale clean air, and your spirits will rise, clearing noxious substances from the mind as well as the body.

A Breathing Checklist

- Take three sets of eight deep breaths (with attendant arm exercises) every morning on arising and in the evening before you go to bed.
- If you're in a sedentary position for over two hours, take four deep breaths as described in exercise 2 on page 176. If you can, stand as you do so.
- In times of stress, either emotional or physical, stop and take several deep breaths. This will slow down your heart rate and help you develop a positive attitude.
- Avoid shallow, rapid breathing.
- As much as possible, stay away from polluted air, including that caused by your own smoking or somebody else's.
- Stay away from grass and trees on which insecticide sprays have been used.
- Integrate deep breathing with yoga sessions—and begin those sessions *today*!

YOGA

When most Americans refer to yoga, they are thinking of hatha yoga, which is mainly physical exercise and postures. (When a friend says, "I'm going to yoga class," he or she almost surely means going to a class in hatha yoga.) But yoga, under its many names and interpretations, is far more a spiritual than a physical discipline, and hatha yoga is only the first step in an eight-step process that leads from self-control and posture through withdrawal from material and sensual desires to an ultimate meditation on and union with the Divine.

Yoga masters practice the discipline throughout their lives, but all of us, through meditation, breathing, physical control, and service to others, can become yoga practitioners, and no better method exists for the release of anxiety and the attainment of serenity. It is a road to health that more and more science-trained doctors, myself definitely included, prescribe.

The word *yoga* is derived from the ancient Sanskrit word *yug,* meaning "a union," in this case a union with the Divine. It is the yoking of the body to the mind, the massage of meditation. It unites body and mind through a series of thoughtful and quiet postures that stimulates the muscles and internal organs and opens our minds to the energy forces of the universe.

In the Eastern tradition, there are seven energy centers called *chakras,* which direct our various emotional and spiritual drives. Yoga realigns and balances the chakras so that the flow of energy can rise unimpeded from the first chakra to the seventh. Yoga is closely associated with meditation, and the combination of the two is a powerful force for wellness.

Yoga and the Lymphatics

Yoga is an ideal tool for lymphatic health. It relaxes the lymph channels and dramatically increases lymph flow through muscular and gravitational pumping of the lymphatic system. The powerful mental images and feeling of peace effected by yoga and meditation release powerful hormonal messengers that dilate and relax the lymphatic channels and increase the clearance of toxic fluids from your body tissues. It is like internal sweating, the "mind's perspiration."

Integral Yoga

Dr. Sandy McLanahan, medical director of the Integral Health Center in Charlottesville, Virginia, and author of *Everyone's Guide to Surgery and Its Natural Alternatives* and *Staying Healthy in the Midst of It All,* feels that yoga is the most powerful tool for treatment of all diseases, including heart disease and cancer. She is involved in Integral Yoga, which is a combination of five practices:

1. Meditation
2. Breathing
3. Stretching
4. Relaxation
5. Serviceful life

Meditation, yoga, breathing, and service to others, all are as important to the maintenance of good health as exercise and diet—and, remarkably, the spiritual life.

Here are some simple yoga positions you can practice by your-self.

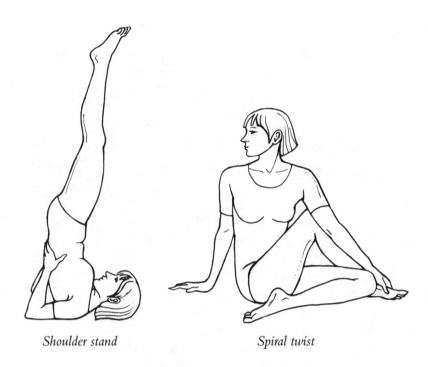

Shoulder stand   Spiral twist

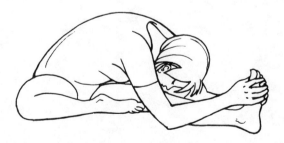

Head to knee

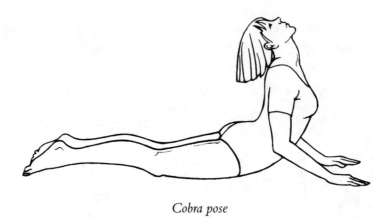

Cobra pose

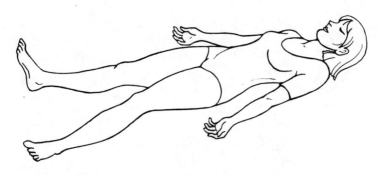

Corpse pose

And here are some "quick chair" yoga exercises you can do at work.

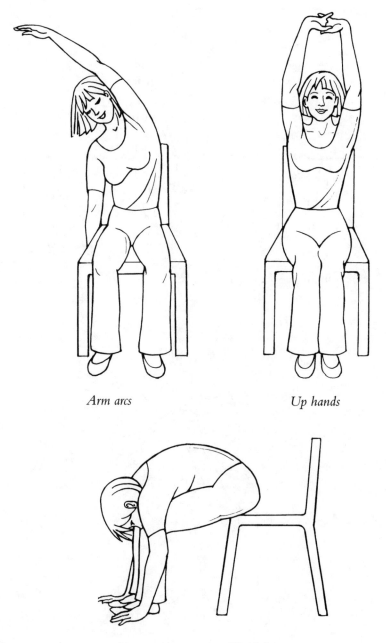

Arm arcs   Up hands

Head down

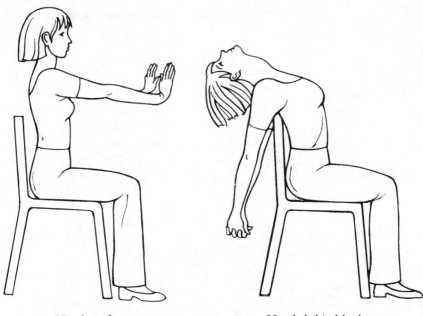

Hands in front   *Hands behind back*

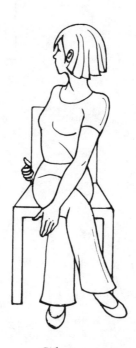

Side turns

Here are twelve basic yoga postures, or asanas, she teaches. If you want fuller information, you can order yoga tapes from the Integral Health Center (1-800-476-1347).

Sun Salutation

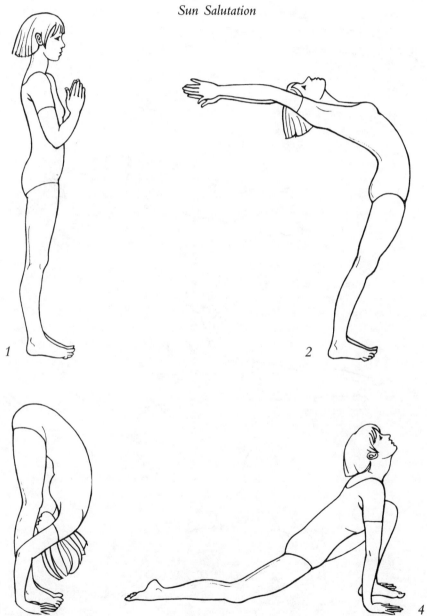

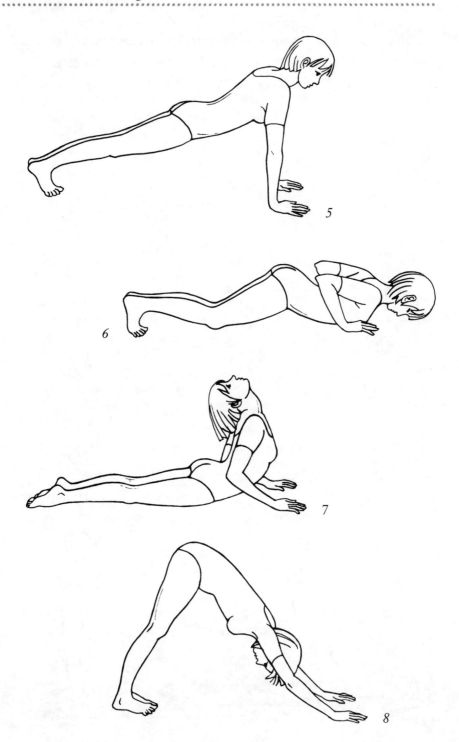

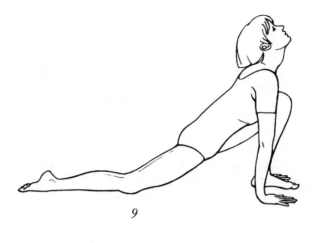

9

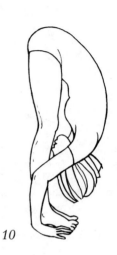

10

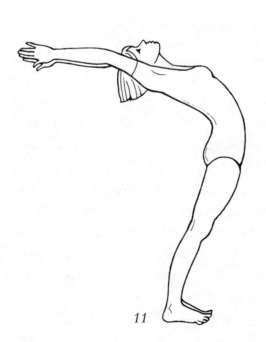

11

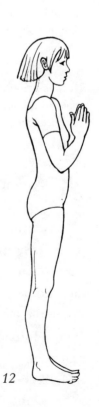

12

9

Spirituality

Man lives in three dimensions: the somatic, the mental, and the spiritual. The spiritual dimension cannot be ignored, for it is what makes us human.

—VIKTOR E. FRANKL, M.D., *The Doctor & the Soul*

Stay awake and keep praying so that you won't come into a crisis. The spirit is eager but the flesh is sick.   —MATTHEW 26:14

This is the great error of our day in the treatment of the human body, that physicians separate the soul from the body.

—HIPPOCRATES, 377 B.C.

Every affection of the mind that is attended with either pain or pleasure, hope or fear, is the cause of an agitation whose influence extends to the heart.   —WILLIAM HARVEY, 1628

Complementary medicine, the kind I advocate and practice, views humankind the way Frankl does, as spirit,
mind, and body. Each of these areas has a profound effect
upon the heart, my area of expertise. The terms *heartbroken* or *sick at heart* are far more than romantic metaphors; they describe a physical condition, even though there may be no viral or bacterial cause.
When the heart is at ease, it is well. When it is dis-eased, the spirit,
mind, and body, either individually or in combination, need to be
addressed.

In Western medicine the body, spirit, and mind have traditionally been segregated. Medicine's focus on the body, how its organs function and its blood flows, ignores the physical effects of the spirit and thus creates a mechanistic view. To many doctors, our bodies are machines to be fixed, not people to be healed. In the seventeenth century, the French philosopher René Descartes concluded that there were two separate substances in the world: matter, which behaved according to physical laws, and spirit, which was dimensionless and immaterial, with an unbridgeable chasm between the two. Body and spirit, brain and mind: these were entities that were distinct and discrete parts of human life and had to be looked at separately.

Descartes's concept dominated medical and religious thought in the following centuries. Western medicine does not treat the inner person; Western religion does not treat the body, only the spirit. Only now are doctors beginning to recognize the enormous role that the spirit, mind, and emotions play in wellness, disease, healing, and the maintenance of health.

While Western thought and practice remained blind to the correlation between spirit and body, other parts of the world knew it all along. Over 4,000 years ago in China, it was noticed that illness followed frustration. The Egyptians in the same period prescribed good cheer and an optimistic attitude as programs for health. The Greeks suggested rest and relaxation for illness, and Galen observed that happy women had less incidence of breast cancer than those who were melancholy. In the biblical book of Proverbs, "a merry heart maketh good medicine."

William James in the nineteenth century and Viktor Frankl in the mid-twentieth both recognized mankind's search for a higher meaning and significance in life. "The pleasure principle might be termed the *will to pleasure*," Frankl writes. "The status drive is equivalent to the *will-to-power*. But where do we hear of that which most deeply inspires man; where is the innate desire to give as much meaning as possible to one's life, to actualize as many values as possible—what I should like to call the *will-to-meaning*?"

The will-to-meaning, he says, is the most human phenomenon of all, since an animal isn't concerned about the meaning of its existence. Yet this life force—for that is exactly what it is—is ironically overlooked by doctors whose purpose it is to maintain a patient's healthy life. Both James and Frankl understood that the brain and the body could be the source of sickness. They saw the lack of spiritual fulfillment as predictive of illness; they understood the power of spirituality, the quest for life's purpose, the vital link between body and soul.

THE NEED FOR SPIRITUAL LIFE

For humankind to be centered, whole, and fulfilled, the spiritual aspect of life must play a role. Whether in the context of organized religion, in support groups without particular religious affiliation, or by following your individual path of meditation and contemplation, some form of spiritual nourishment and solace is necessary. There is empirical evidence.

Separate studies by doctors Larry Dossey and Rudolph Byrd demonstrated that prayer can facilitate healing. Other studies at Duke University demonstrated that people who regularly attended church had a better immune system with higher levels of T, helper, and killer cells than those who did not. A study of patients with a religious background showed a lower diastolic blood pressure, fewer admissions to the hospital, less coronary vascular disease, and fewer complications in cardiac catheterizations than in the general population. A study of 10,000 male civil servants in Israel showed that, independent of lifestyle, religious orthodoxy lowered the risk of coronary heart disease.

When 230 patients over fifty-five years old were studied by Oxman in 1995, those deriving no comfort, sustenance, or strength from religious beliefs had over a threefold increased mortality following open heart surgery. In 1990, Levin and Vanderpool demonstrated a significant relationship between low incidence of cardiovascular disease and high level of spiritual practice.

In a 1991 meta-analysis of twenty-seven studies, Larsen found that twenty-two of them showed a positive relationship between health and religious commitment. Heart disease, hypertension, and overall mortality were improved by going to church. In a classic study, George W. Comstock and Kay B. Partridge offered compelling evidence for the beneficial association between church attendance and heart disease.

According to an October 1994 survey of hospitalized patients, 98 percent believed in God and almost as many had a conviction that spiritual and physical well-being were equally important; 75 percent prayed daily and felt their spiritual needs should be addressed by their physicians; 48 percent wanted their physicians' prayers.

Some doctors, like my son-in-law Mehmet Oz, bring faith healers into the operating room with them; others make sure that their patients are seen by a spiritual counselor before and after major surgery. Mehmet, a Harvard-trained cardiac surgeon, started the Complementary Care Center at Columbia Presbyterian Hospital in New York, where he uses therapeutic touch, aroma therapy, and hypnosis on his heart transplant and surgical patients.

Many of the doctors at Johns Hopkins Hospital pray with their patients (including the legendary brain surgeon Benjamin Carson), and at the huge statue of Christ in its main rotunda hundreds of religious messages are left in support of the patients, not only by their families but by doctors and nurses as well.

I cite all these examples simply to show that science can be applied even to so mystical a facet of our beings as spirituality. A deep belief in some higher power or cosmological force, whether it be God (of any denomination) or a simple belief in human goodness and the capacity to love, is a factor in good health and rapid recovery. One must go outside oneself, see oneself in the context of the universe, be able to love, care for, and give to others. This is one way to physical health.

SPIRITUAL HEALING

Daniel J. Benor defined spiritual healing as the intentional influence of one or more people on another living system without the use of any known physical means of intervention. Some individuals can, with greater difficulty, do this for themselves. Spiritual intervention, Benor goes on to say, is nonlocal; that is, not necessarily confined to the present moment or locality. Doctors at Johns Hopkins Hospital, for instance, encourage a patient's family to set up prayer groups in their hometown while the operation is going on in Baltimore, and at Duke University, concrete evidence has been shown of the effectiveness of such distant healing.

If the patient is able to participate, so much the better. Rudolph Byrd conducted a double-blind, randomized study on the effects of prayer on coronary care patients. At the end of ten months, the group being prayed for required fewer diuretics and antibiotics and less ventilator assistance than the control group.

LOVE, FORGIVENESS, AND HOPE

It has been known for years that negative emotions are strong predictors of heart disease and other chronic degenerative diseases. What is not so well known but is becoming increasingly evident is that *positive* emotions such as love, forgiveness, self-esteem, optimism, and hope can help prevent disease and even restore health after an illness. Indeed, in a recent study by Helgeson and Fritz of patients who had undergone successful angioplasty, patients who scored high in positive emotions and feelings were three times less likely than those who scored low to sustain a new coronary event.

You can see negative versus positive emotions at work in yourself. The next time you feel anger, hatred, or pessimism, try to become aware of your body. Your muscles will be tight, particularly in your upper back and neck; your breathing will be shallow; your stomach will churn. There is quite the opposite result if you can genuinely say, "I love you" or "I forgive you" or "I have hope." Your body feels lighter; the muscles relax; your breath is deep and regular—you're hungry!

It's more difficult to discern emotion if it's been hidden within your body, sometimes since childhood. Yet resentments fester; swallowed anger can lodge in your stomach; parental belittling when you're a child can affect your posture and self-esteem as an adult; a life seared by unhappiness can determine the way you walk and talk and breathe. You may not be conscious of your feelings; they may be so embedded that they seem natural. If they're pointed out by a therapist or friend, often the response is disbelief or denial. But the feelings are there nevertheless, and—usually with the aid of a therapist but sometimes on one's own—they can be changed.

A man I know was burdened by memories of his mother—long since dead—who had constantly criticized him when he was a child. He professed great love for her, said he thought of her and missed her every day, yet he walked with a stoop, his eyes were constantly downcast, he was constantly sick, he was unable to establish any long-term romantic relationship, and he had not lived up to his professional potential.

I advised him to see a therapist.

"Does your mother still live with you?" the therapist asked in an early session.

"Yes. She's part of me. She's in my memory, in my heart."

"Does she pay you rent?"

My friend looked up, startled.

"Rent? Of course not! She's dead."

"Well," the therapist said, "if she doesn't pay rent, you should evict her."

It was, my friend said, an epiphany that changed his life. Evict her he did, and he began to live.

THERAPEUTIC TECHNIQUES

A variety of therapies designed to change emotional and spiritual outlook have become popular over the past two decades, and in each case there is ample testimony to their effectiveness.

Cognitive Behavioral Therapy

Cognitive behavioral therapy focuses on influencing behavior through changing the patient's thinking processes. There are beneficial cardiovascular effects through positive modifications in relationships, smoking, medications, diet, and hostile behavior.

Music Therapy

That music calms, soothes, and inspires the spirit is indisputable. For some it is a means of sharpening the creative urge and imagination, for others a way to relax or a spur to meditation. Yet as Don Campbell points out in his book *The Mozart Effect,* music can have positive—some might say amazing—health benefits as well. Therapists at Beth Abraham, a hospital affiliated with New York's Albert Einstein College of Medicine, have shown that music is a key to gaining access to memories; that it can aid in the reversal or prevention of certain types of deafness; and that it aids in the recovery of neural function by promoting nerve cell regeneration, by establishing new neural connections and pathways, and by shortening the time to recovery of function. "Scientists," Campbell writes, "have known that compensatory mechanisms can be triggered by loss of neurologic function. Parts of the brain that have lain dormant can 'take over,' in whole or part, the damaged function. . . . This phenomenon may be jump-started or kicked into higher gear by music and sound, as well as by certain types of exercise and language."

Music has been shown to produce great results in the operating room, both in easing the patient's anxiety and in drowning out distracting noise and potentially bothersome conversation. And as Campbell points out, music is used in a variety of hospitals for a variety of reasons: to reduce complications and speed recovery after anesthesia (London's Charing Cross Hospital) and aid in such areas as physical rehabilitation, respiratory intensive care, breast cancer support groups, stroke recovery, labor and deliveries, even psychiatry (St. Luke's Hospital in Chesterfield, Missouri). At the University of Massachusetts Medical Center, harp music has been prescribed in place of tranquilizers and painkillers for cancer patients, and the University of Louisville School of Medicine has reported success with the use of music for patients with Alzheimer's.

Clearly there is a physiological response to music that goes well beyond the auditory, but we have not been able to pinpoint exactly how and why it functions. Still, music has been used for centuries both to incite (the drums of Africa, the bugles of Western armies) and to soothe. In *The Magic Flute*, the hero, Tamino, tames wild animals with his music. It can tame us as well.

Imagery Therapy

When the wife of a good friend of mine developed a glioblas-
toma—a kind of brain cancer that is nearly always fatal—she went
to a support group where they practiced imaging, seeing mental
pictures of healthy cells devouring the unhealthy ones. The technique did not cure her, and there is no evidence that the cancer
cells were any fewer, but the imaging provided her with enormous
solace, for she felt she was working alongside her doctors to battle
the disease.

Imagery therapy attempts to heal by evocation of the senses
through the use of imagination. It is an age-old therapy long used
by medicine men and shamans in healing rites, orchestrating the
connection between the body's movements, perceptions, and emotions. It has been shown to reduce metabolic rate, heart rate, and
blood pressure. Often, videotapes, spoken cassettes, or a live facilita-
tor can help the patient maintain concentration and strengthen
technique.

Laughter Therapy

Norman Cousins's *Anatomy of an Illness,* which described his miracle cure through the use of laughter induced by watching Marx
Brothers movies, only made explicit a phenomenon known about
for centuries. Indeed, in the 1600s, Sir Thomas Sydenham said that
"the arrival of a good clown exercises a more beneficial influence
upon the health of a town than the arrival of twenty asses laden
with drugs." Laughter increases immunity through the production
of killer cells and T cells and the suppression of the sympathetic
nervous system. By changing the psychological environment,
laughter creates an atmosphere of relaxation and calmness. It
delights me to think that Robin Williams or Richard Pryor has had

a greater impact on the nation's health than any number of gray-faced doctors prescribing Xanax or Percocet.

Hypnosis

Medical hypnosis is far different from the hypnosis practiced by magicians for the entertainment of their audience. Doctors and psychologists have used it therapeutically as anesthesia and to unlock emotional inhibitions that damage the body as well as the mind, and the results have been extraordinary.

Timeshifting

Often overlooked as a factor in healing and spirituality is time itself. Yet, as Dr. Stephan Rechtschaffen has shown, time has many speeds, and one's relation to it must be varied. To you, nine seconds might seem not enough to do anything significant; to Michael Jordan (it is he who used the example), it is ample to bring a ball up court, see the position of every player, and shoot a winning basket. All of us have complained about "not having enough hours in the day." Yet in fact there are plenty of hours, and if we use them all for work, we are *mis*using them.

If we all learn to slow down in our ever faster paced world of cell phones, faxes, E-mail, and Internet—if we can take some time for meditation (even for ten minutes in the car during the time between arriving home and opening your front door), for quiet walks, for listening to music, for an unplanned vacation during a weekend or even an afternoon—our spiritual life will flourish. We must learn to control time rather than letting it control us; we must bend it to the needs of our psyche as well as to our material well-being. It was Lucretius who wrote, "It is great wealth for a man to live sparingly with a calm mind."

MEDICINE OF THE MIND

All these therapies, and others involving sound, dance, painting, and other mind-body techniques, have to do with the mind—that part of you which can reach the realm of spiritual investigation and fulfillment—and not the brain, which is concerned with rational thought. If the mind is calm, the body is calm, and as Herbert Benson, who did groundbreaking work on the relaxation response, shows, when the body is at ease, blood pressure, heart rate, and breathing rate decrease. As we've seen, the meditative mind cannot be in distress.

Spirituality often requires a change in mind-set. If you're rushed, burdened with work, filled with concern about family, money, a relationship, a job, you will have little place for peace of mind. Similarly, if you're angry, depressed, worried, scattered, or anxious, there's no room for ease of spirit. I recognize that it's a lot simpler to tell yourself to calm down than it is to *be* calm, but even without the aid of a therapist, here are a few ways to go about the change. (I know I've briefly mentioned some of them before, but they bear elaboration.)

- Create a special place—a "sacred space"—in which to meditate or practice any of the other mind-altering techniques. It can be a chapel, a closet, or even a corner of a room that is marked off in your mind as a place to center yourself and contemplate less mundane and more profound things.
- Think optimistically rather than pessimistically. The deal *will* go through. The relationship *will* endure. Your children *will* get over it (whatever "it" is). If you use optimism as a mantra, it will in time become second nature, part of your psychic makeup.
- Be positive. This is a corollary to optimism, a way of looking at a

task or event in the best light. The simple attitude "I can do it" is as or more important to success (and I don't mean only material success) as careful advance planning.

- Set positive goals—again, not only in the realm of material goods. Many people lead their lives and arrange their thoughts simply to avoid failure. Indeed, they may not fail—but they will surely not succeed.

- Practice positive visualization. We've talked about visualization as a factor in cure. But it can also be used by the healthy to further the achievement of goals and as an aid to optimism. If you set a definite positive goal for the future (a new house in five years; a better family life; a real relationship with God), it will come to pass if you can *see* it (the house has rooms and furniture, the family is together at dinner, your God comes to you in church). The more specific the details, the better.

- Become aware of self-talk. Perpetual use of the *I* word, as former President George Bush has pointed out, can lead to a self-involvement that excludes others from your thought. Narcissism virtually guarantees small-mindedness, for it limits the world to yourself and makes it impossible to think of others. The self-involved are rarely involved with higher concepts and ideals, and certainly not with spirituality, which presupposes a force far greater than the self.

- Ask better questions: not questions that debunk, satirize, or are meant to show off but ones that take the inquiry into account, respect opposing viewpoints, and attempt to broaden your knowledge. You must also ask questions about the *why* of things, the relation of yourself to the Grand Design, metaphysical questions that mankind has been struggling with since thought began. These questions are the paving stones of the spiritual road. They lead, in the Buddhist sense, to Enlightenment.

- Laugh. You can, as Norman Cousins did, watch funny movies, listen to comedy tapes, tell and enjoy jokes. But mishaps can also be funny. The ability to laugh at yourself is a rare and valuable asset. Life is at once sublime and ridiculous. An ironic attitude is often more healing than a sentimental one. We are God's creatures. God gave us laughter, and we should use it to the fullest.

THE "NEW AGE" DOCTOR

I am one of the many physicians who believe both in orthodox cardiology—indeed, we are now at the point that it has become an exact science—and in complementary medicine. As I read over this chapter, I'm struck by what the medical establishment might have thought of it as recently as five years ago. But New Age thinking (a misnomer if there ever was one; the ideas were propounded in Asia before Egyptian civilization was born) has joined with scientific thinking, spirituality with up-to-date medical technology.

As I turn to how my program can be modified for specific diseases, remember that the ideal healing method incorporates both the wisdom of the ancient East and the know-how of modern Western science.

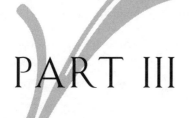

PART III

*Program
Modification for
Specific Diseases*

B efore I come to specific recommendations for specific diseases, there are a few more general precepts to point out about integrative medicine.

1. The body has natural abilities for homeostasis and healing.
2. Natural remedies often have the desired outcome without the significant side effects that may accompany the use of drugs.
3. The human being is a complex combination of spirit, mind, and body—all of which can contribute to health. The doctor's aim is to see the patient as a whole.
4. Social and environmental conditions must be taken into consideration.
5. Symptoms are guideposts to the root causes of disease and therefore should be treated but not silenced.
6. Patients should be encouraged to become participants in their recoveries.
7. Each patient is an individual and must be treated individually.

10

Heart Disease

HEART DISEASE, ANGINA, AND HEART ATTACK

Coronary artery disease is a form of arteriosclerosis, a hardening of the coronary arteries that supply the heart muscle. (Arteriosclerosis also occurs in other arteries of the body, such as the brain, which can result in a stroke.) The buildup of cholesterol, calcium, and clotting in the artery limits blood flow and prevents oxygen from being delivered to the tissue. If the heart doesn't receive enough oxygen, the patient experiences pain—called *angina*—in the chest, arms, or jaw. Angina is a warning signal and is not necessarily accompanied by damage to the heart muscle. Generally it lasts no more than ten minutes and is relieved by rest. If heart muscle damage *has* occurred, however, the process is called a *myocardial infarction,* or heart attack.

The risk of coronary artery disease is increased by smoking, obesity, high blood pressure, diabetes, lack of physical activity, high blood cholesterol, and stress or tension. I've shown how lack of exercise, improper breathing, and a high-fat diet make heart disease more likely, and I've recommended a program to lessen the risk.

But what if you already have coronary heart disease or angina or have experienced a heart attack? First and foremost, it is *vital* that you continue to see your doctor regularly (or, in the case of angina, that you see your doctor immediately, even though the pain will have passed). *Do not self-diagnose! Do not self-medicate!* Heart problems of any kind are potentially life-and-death circumstances, and to ignore the signals or to assume that because the pain has stopped you are "better" is to play Russian roulette.

Initially, the standard treatment for angina or a coronary episode includes:

- Medications to decrease the oxygen need of the heart
- Mild blood thinners such as aspirin
- A low-fat diet identical or similar to the one I have described, with the addition of the vitamins and supplements listed later (page 207)
- The strict elimination of risk factors such as high blood pressure, high blood sugar, high LDL, smoking, and obesity

If these don't eliminate the symptoms, or if you are in a life-threatening situation, your doctor may suggest an angioplasty, a procedure that stretches open the blocked vessels, or even open-heart surgery to bypass the blockage. These technological marvels are by now routine and very safe. If it turns out that you need such surgery, your chances of coming through it unscathed are over 98 percent.

Still, it's better if you don't get that far. Several studies have shown that stress reduction, exercise, and proper diet can be used in combination to treat coronary artery disease with dramatic success.

In fact, these measures have been successful in *reversing* coronary heart disease. You get better without the use of a knife.

Basic Healthy Heart Program

Along with my Fourteen-Day Diet for lymphatic health, I recommend taking the following vitamins and minerals. (Many of them are also beneficial in the prevention of heart disease.) *I also recommend certain brand names based on their uniformity, quality, and long-standing reputation. I have no financial interest or consulting arrangement with any of these companies.*

- High-potency vitamin and mineral containing at least 50 mg B complex (Solgar VM 75). Note: Men or post-menopausal women should take the formula without iron.
- *Vitamin C:* 1,000 mg twice a day (such as Ester C, ascorbic acid, or calcium ascorbate). Note: Vitamin C enhances the effectiveness of vitamin E, strengthens the walls of arteries, lessens the risk of blood clots, and can raise the level of HDLs.
- *Vitamin E:* 400 to 800 IU daily. In presence of hypertension or diabetes, begin with 100 IU daily and increase. Note: Vitamin E decreases the "stickiness" of platelets, the blood cells that cause blood clots.

If you are taking anticoagulants, please check with your physician. High dosages of vitamin C and vitamin E may alter the effect of warfarin (Coumadin).

- *Vitamin B_6:* 50 mg daily. Note: Vitamin B_6 breaks down homocysteine.

- *Folic acid:* 400 mcg. Note: Folic acid breaks down homo-cysteine.
- *Vitamin B$_{12}$:* 1 mg sublingual daily
- *Vitamin B$_1$:* 200 mg daily, if taking furosemide or other diuretics
- *Magnesium citrate* (Twin Labs): 400 to 800 mg daily. (Magnesium in higher doses can cause diarrhea. If this occurs, titrate to tolerance.) In the absence of kidney failure, slowly increase to 800 mg in divided doses.
- *Calcium citrate* (Twin Labs): 500 mg twice daily. Note: Calcium, magnesium, and selenium all play major roles in heart health. Magnesium, for example, can prevent irregular heart rhythms and dilate blood vessels to improve circulation. Low levels of selenium have been associated with heart disease and an increased risk of heart attack.

Calcium and magnesium may be taken in a combination product.

- *Chromium:* 200 mcg daily
- *Zinc:* 15 to 30 mg daily. Check your multivitamin to see if it contains zinc. Do not exceed 30 mg.
- *Copper:* 2 to 3 mg daily
- *Selenium:* 200 mcg daily taken with vitamin E
- *Fish oils:* EFA/DHA: 3 g daily, or flaxseed oil: 1 tablespoon daily. Note: Omega-3 thins the blood, thus reducing the chance of blood clots.
- *Coenzyme Q$_{10}$* (CoQ$_{10}$): as a soft gel, 60 mg twice a day. Higher doses are needed for specific conditions such as congestive heart failure or cardiomyopathy. Do not abruptly cease taking CoQ$_{10}$, taper off gradually. Note: Coenzyme Q$_{10}$ is found chiefly in the heart muscle and is used regularly in Japan for treating heart diseases. It assists

with energy production in the heart muscle and has been shown to lessen the frequency of angina attacks.

- *Garlic* (Garlitrin 4000): 4,000 mcg as tablets or capsules with allicin or eaten fresh. Note: Garlic counters the blood's tendency to clot following a high-fat meal.

Exercise

As we've seen, exercise is one of the prime factors in warding off heart disease. It is equally or even more important *after* heart disease, but it is essential that you develop a new exercise program with your doctor. Simply going back to the Exercycle or treadmill and resuming your preattack routine can be fatal.

A Vitamin and Mineral Plan for Angina and Heart Disease

Again, do not use this program without guidance from your doctor. If your doctor is uninformed about vitamins and minerals, as many doctors are, then consult a nutritionist. The following is a highly effective program for many sufferers but by no means all. Pain and disease are as individual as fingerprints. Experimentation with dosages will probably be required until the right levels are reached. To the Basic Healthy Heart Program, add or increase to the following:

Supplements

- *N-acetylcysteine:* 600 mg 3 times daily
- *Coenzyme Q_{10}:* increase to 60 mg 3 times daily. Do not abruptly withdraw CoQ_{10}. If discontinued, taper off gradually.

- *L-carnitine:* 500 to 1,000 mg 2 times daily, away from meals
- *Pantethine:* 300 mg 3 times daily
- *L-lysine:* 5 g daily, away from meals
- *Hawthorn berry:* 80 mg 2 times daily, standardized to 15 mg of procyanidin oligomers per 80 mg capsules. Can potentiate digitalis. Use under the care of your health professional.
- *Fish oils:* EFA/DHA, increasing to 2,000 mg 3 times daily. Dietary fatty fish consumption may be increased instead.
- *Alpha lipoic acid:* 50 mg daily, may be doubled under physician's supervision.

Note

- In higher doses, fish oils and vitamin E can prolong bleeding.
- Unless specified, all supplements are taken with meals.

Avoid

- Caffeine in all forms: coffee, tea, colas, and chocolate
- Sugar

Increase

- Fatty fish consumption: salmon, cod, tuna, sardines, mackerel, etc.

Exercise

- Follow physician's recommendation.

CONGESTIVE HEART FAILURE

When the heart cannot function normally as a pump, sending blood throughout the body, the resulting very serious condition is known as congestive heart failure. Without blood flow, vital organs do not function properly. Ankles and legs swell. Fluid accumulates in the lungs, causing shortness of breath.

Congestive heart failure is most commonly caused by arteriosclerosis, which results in a lack of blood supply to the heart. Other causes include high blood pressure, congenital heart disease, heart valve disease, heart attack, and emphysema. It is most commonly experienced as breathlessness, especially with mild exertion such as climbing a flight of stairs or when lying down. Fatigue is also present, with or without chest pain. There may be loss of appetite, the need to urinate frequently during the night, and mental confusion.

Only your doctor can diagnose and treat congestive heart failure. He or she will probably prescribe several medications, including diuretics or water pills, beta-blockers, and so-called ACE inhibitors, all of which work to reduce the work of the heart, and digitalis and other drugs to increase the strength of the heart muscle.

Diet After Congestive Heart Failure

My Fourteen-Day Diet for lymphatic health, being low in salt, is a fine starting point. As for supplements, CoQ_{10} has been used with dramatic effect. L-carnitine, and amino acid, has also been shown to be beneficial since it appears to help the heart muscle cells produce energy more efficiently. Magnesium can prevent irregular heart rhythms, which are particularly to be avoided in those with congestive heart failure. Vitamin E can be helpful for its anticlotting effects.

Your diet should be carefully worked out with your doctor, or with a skilled nutritionist if you feel your doctor is not knowledgeable enough in this area. It is possible, for example, that you may want a diet even lower in salt than the one I recommend. You should also heed your doctor's recommendations on exercise, for the type and amount depend upon the diagnosis and severity of the disease. I've seen heart patients begin to exercise and return to work too early, often, alas, with fatal results.

A Vitamin and Mineral Plan for Congestive Heart Failure

Use under the supervision of your health-care professional.

DO NOT SELF-DIAGNOSE.
DO NOT SELF-MEDICATE.

To the Basic Healthy Heart Program, add or increase the following:

VITAMINS
- *Vitamin C:* increase to 1,000 mg 3 times daily

AMINO ACIDS
- *L-carnitine:* up to 500 mg 3 times daily, away from food
- *L-taurine:* 2,000 mg 2 to 3 times daily in divided doses
- *L-arginine:* 2,000 to 4,000 mg at bedtime. May be increased by your physician.

OTHERS
- *Coenzyme Q$_{10}$:* as soft gel, 200 to 400 mg daily in divided doses. Do not abruptly withdraw CoQ$_{10}$. If discontinued, taper gradually.
- *Ribose:* 1 to 5 g daily

HERBS
- *Hawthorn berry:* 80 mg 2 times daily, standardized to 15 mg of procyanidin oligomers per 80 mg capsules. Can potentiate digitalis. Use carefully under the care of your health professional.
- *Ginkgo biloba:* 60 mg 2 times daily

NOTES
- Ginkgo biloba can thin the blood.
- Unless specified, all supplements are taken with meals.

EXERCISE
- Follow your physician's recommendations.

A Vitamin and Mineral Plan for Cardiac Arrhythmias

To the Basic Healthy Heart Program, add or increase to the following:

SUPPLEMENTS
- In the absence of kidney failure, slowly increase magnesium citrate to 800 mg in divided doses. Calcium citrate remains at 1,000 mg.
- *L-taurine:* 3 g daily
- *Coenzyme Q$_{10}$:* higher ranges up to 300 mg daily. Do not abruptly withdraw CoQ$_{10}$. If discontinued, taper gradually.

- *Hawthorn berry:* 80 to 250 mg 2 times daily. Standardized to 15 mg of procyanidin oligomers per 80 mg capsules. Can potentiate digitalis. Use under the care of your health professional.
- *Potassium:* eat potassium-rich food. If not possible, supplementation is available: 100 mg daily. See note below on renal failure.
- *Fish oils:* EFA/DHA, increasing to 2,000 mg 3 times daily. Resume 1,000 mg 3 times daily when desired results are achieved.

NOTES

- In higher doses, fish oils and vitamin E can prolong bleeding.
- Renal failure patients should consult their physicians.
- Unless specified, all supplements are taken with meals.
- In lieu of fish oil, use 1 tablespoon cod liver oil with orange juice once a day.

A Vitamin and Mineral Plan for Lowering Cholesterol Without Drugs

To the Basic Health Heart Program add or increase to the following:

SUPPLEMENTS

- *Vitamin C:* increase to 1,000 mg 3 times daily
- *No-flush niacin* (inositol hexaniacinate): 500 mg 2 times daily for 2 weeks, then increase to 1,000 mg 3 times daily. While taking high doses of niacin, liver profiles must be checked every three months. With diabetes, do not use niacin. Replace with Pantethine (see below).

- *Gugulipid:* Standardized extract of 25 mg per 500 mg tablet 3 times daily
- *Chromium picolinate:* 200 mcg 2 times daily, reduce to 200 daily after desired results are achieved
- *Garlic:* Eat plenty of fresh garlic or garlic tablets or capsules with allicin; potential of 4,000 mcg, 1 tablet daily

NOTES
- High-dose garlic can potentiate warfarin.
- If, after six weeks, levels have not sufficiently lowered, add:
  —*L-carnitine:* 500 mg 3 times daily, between meals
  —*Pantethine:* 300 mg 3 times daily
- Unless specified, all supplements are taken with meals.

DIET
- Emphasize soluble fiber: oat bran, barley, apple and grapefruit pectin, and guar gum.
- Increase soy.
- Eat generous amounts of fresh garlic, or double amount taken, or take a capsule.
- Include: Flaxseed oil, 1 tablespoon daily in juice or in salads. Use small amounts of olive oil for sautéing and dressing salads.
- Exclude: Meat, dairy products, processed foods such as refined flours and cereals, margarine, any foods containing partially hydrogenated vegetable oils, sugars, peanuts, peanut butter, and peanut oil.

EXERCISE
- Regular exercise—1 hour daily under physician's supervision.

LIFESTYLE
- Stress modification: Consciously observe negative emotion—replace with positive response. Learn how to meditate, use visualization, and learn how to breathe. Yoga relaxes the mind and the body. Biofeedback for those who desire a "high tech" modality.

A Vitamin and Mineral Plan for Lowering Homocysteine

To the Basic Healthy Heart Program add or increase to the following:

VITAMINS
- *Vitamin B$_6$:* 50 mg daily
- *Folic acid:* 1 to 1.6 mg daily
- *Vitamin B$_{12}$:* 1,000 mcg sublingual daily
- *Trimethylglycine:* 750 mg tablet 2 times daily, away from meals

NOTES
- When homocysteine has been lowered, omit extra B$_6$, reduce folic acid to 400 mcg, and reduce trimethylglycine to 1 tablet daily.
- Unless specified, all supplements are taken with meals.

A Vitamin and Mineral Plan for Lowering Triglycerides

To the Basic Healthy Heart Program add or increase to the following:

SUPPLEMENTS
- *Pantethine:* 300 mg 3 times daily
- *Chromium picolinate:* 200 mcg 3 times daily

- *Gugulipid:* (standardized to 25 mg of gugulsterone per 500 mg tablet) 1 tablet 3 times daily
- *L-carnitine:* 500 mg 3 times daily, between meals
- Increase garlic

NOTES
- High doses of garlic can potentiate warfarin.
- Unless specified, all supplements are taken with meals.
- In higher doses, fish oils and vitamin E can prolong bleeding.

DIET
- Normalize weight.
- Reduce fruit consumption. Avoid fruit juices, alcohol, and all sugars.
- **Avoid refined carbohydrates: refined flour—white bread, white pasta, white rice, cookies, and cakes.**
- **Avoid high-glycemic foods: carrots, corn, and potatoes.**
- Increase soy.
- Increase garlic.
- Increase fish oils: EFA/DHA increase to 2 g 3 times daily or eat cold water fatty fish 4 times weekly (salmon, cod, tuna, sardines, mackerel, etc.).

EXERCISE
- Follow your physician's recommendations.

LIFESTYLE
- Follow your physician's recommendations.

11

Cancer

I have said little about cancer earlier in this book, so let me
begin here with an overview.

Cancer has four general categories depending on what area
of the body is affected: *lymphomas* develop from the lymphatic system; *leukemias* are blood cancers; *sarcomas* are cancers in the bone,
soft tissue, muscle, and connective tissues; and *carcinomas*, the most
common forms, are cancers of the glands, skin, mucous membranes,
and various organs. All cancers do not form or progress at the same
speed; prostate cancer, for example, is particularly slow moving. But
all cancers are cells "gone wild" in the body. If untreated, they grow
uncontrollably, often long before you are aware they exist. These
abnormal cells develop their own network of blood vessels for support and eventually form a tumor. The cancer takes its nourishment
from the body itself. If left unchecked, most cancers will metastasize
and spread to other areas of the body.

One out of every three people will develop cancer over a lifetime. Over half a million Americans die from cancer each year. Every minute someone dies from cancer; every day, 1,400. This year—2000—cancer is expected to overtake heart disease as the number one cause of death in the United States.

CANCER PREVENTION

Yes, this chapter concerns a specific micronutrient program for cancer patients, with emphasis on breast and colon cancer, but it's worth reiterating that my Fourteen-Day Diet for lymphatic health is the best place to begin the *prevention* process. Being high in fiber means that it combats colon cancer. Stressing high quantities of fruits and vegetables means that if you follow it, you reduce your risk of cancer by *one half.* (This is particularly true for cancer of the breast, colon, lung, cervix, stomach, esophagus, bladder, pancreas, ovary, and oral cavity.) And it contains all the foods now being studied for their anticancer properties, such as garlic, onions, ginger, soybeans, licorice, carrots, green tea, turmeric, citrus fruits, tomatoes, potatoes, broccoli, cauliflower, brussels sprouts, brown rice, flaxseed, barley, shiitake mushrooms, a variety of leafy vegetables, and yogurt. This means that not only will you reduce your risk of cancer, you will be abetting your overall health (deliciously).

Here are fourteen ways to avoid cancer:

1. Follow the Fourteen-Day Diet for lymphatic health.
2. Avoid excess alcohol, which can play a role in cancers of the liver, mouth, stomach, and esophagus.
3. Avoid excess iron. Do not take additional iron unless blood tests show you are deficient.
4. Drink spring or filtered water. Chlorinated water has been linked to bladder cancer.

5. Avoid artificial sweeteners, food additives, and artificial colors and flavors.

6. *Do not smoke.* Besides lung cancer, which accounts for about one-fifth of all cancer deaths, smoking is linked to cancers of the esophagus, larynx, mouth, pancreas, kidney, and bladder.

7. Avoid exposure to harmful chemicals. They are in our air, water, food, medicines, and cleaning products. Take stock of your environment and eliminate as many poisons as possible.

8. Avoid overexposure to ultraviolet radiation from the sun.

9. When you're outdoors, particularly on the beach, use sunscreen.

10. Avoid exposure to harmful radiation in X rays.

11. Detect and then avoid electromagnetic fields in your home.

12. Exercise.

13. Maintain an optimistic outlook and "feed" the body positive thoughts.

14. Follow regular spiritual practice.

BREAST CANCER

One in nine women will develop breast cancer in her lifetime. Yet while we have spent billions on new methods of detection and treatment, the sad fact is that the death rate from breast cancer has not been dramatically decreased: on the contrary, the occurrence has increased dramatically. Again, *prevention* is where we should be turning our attention.

Once more, the Fourteen-Day Diet for lymphatic health is the place to start, particularly concentrating on green tea, cruciferous vegetables such as cabbage, broccoli, and cauliflower, and foods high in beta-carotene such as yellow and orange fruits and vegetables, as well as soy products, garlic, and onions. Bok choy, kale, and mustard and turnip greens also have protective properties. At the Institute for Hormone Research in New York City, studies show that substance in these vegetables called *indoles* have the ability to affect estrogen metabolism in such a way as to lower the risk of breast cancer.

Obesity, total caloric intake, and lack of dietary fiber have been associated with breast cancer (fiber through its effect on estrogen metabolism). Lack of selenium is also a factor. Ohio, having the lowest percentage of selenium in the soil, has the highest breast cancer rate, while South Dakota, with selenium-rich soil, has the lowest incidence. Iodine is another mineral that, if deficient, may be related to breast cancer, which is why my diet includes shellfish, sea vegetables, kelp, and iodized salt. Studies done in Japan after World War II showed that miso, a fermented soy paste, is a cancer preventive. Current studies have demonstrated the same effects for soybeans, tempeh, and textured soy protein, all of which lower estrogen levels and protect DNA from mutation.

Vitamins, too, play an important part. Researchers at the National Cancer Institute of Canada showed that vitamin C was the most protective. As reported by Jean Carper in *Food—Your Miracle Medicine,* "Eating too little vitamin C was more critical than eating too much fat." The researchers concluded that by adding 380 milligrams of vitamin C a day, the risk of breast cancer would drop by 16 percent in all women and in postmenopausal women by 24 percent.

Vitamin D, which is produced by sunlight, may offer some protection against breast cancer, particularly in postmenopausal women, and dramatic results have been reported from a Danish study, admittedly small, for CoQ_{10}.

Regular exercise is a known preventive since it reduces estrogen levels. A study at Harvard's Center for Population Studies found that in over 5,000 college graduates, former athletes had half the rate of breast cancer of their nonathletic counterparts. And here again, a positive attitude seems to have a direct bearing on reducing the risk of breast cancer.

Supplement Plan for Breast Cancer Prevention

High-potency multivitamin and mineral: VM 75 (Solgar), with iron for premenopausal women, without iron for men and postmenopausal women, 1 tablet daily

Vitamin C: as ascorbic acid, calcium ascorbate, or Ester C, 1 g 3 times daily. Higher doses for treatment.

Vitamin D: 400 IU daily (added to the 400 IU in most multivitamins). This equals 800 IU daily, which is well within safe levels. There is a vitamin-D deficiency in the United States, especially among older people in the north. If taking cod liver oil, omit this vitamin supplement.

Vitamin E: 400 IU daily. In the presence of hypertension, diabetes, or rheumatic heart disease, begin with 100 IU daily and increase to 400 IU daily over six weeks.

Calcium citrate plus magnesium (Twin Labs): 2 with breakfast, 2 with lunch, 4 at bedtime

Zinc: 20 mg daily. Check your multivitamin to see if it contains zinc. Do not exceed 30 mg.

Copper: 2 mg daily

Selenium (Twin Labs): 200 mcg daily. Take with vitamin E.

Bioflavonoids: 1,000 mg three times daily

Astragalus: as directed on label

Garlic extract: (Garlitrin 4000): 1 daily

Green magnum or kyro greens: in juice as directed on label

CoQ$_{10}$ (soft gel): 100 mg 2 times daily. Higher doses for
   treatment.

Quercetin: 1 capsule (150 mg) daily

Flaxseed oil (Barleans): 1 to 2 tablespoons daily. Refrigerate,
   do not heat, and use within three months. Or ground
   flaxseed, 1 to 2 tablespoons on cereal or in juice.

Shark cartilage (Benefin): for treatment of breast cancer as
   directed on label or as directed by your heath-care professional.

Reminder: Unless specified, all vitamin and mineral supplements should be taken just before or after a meal.

This program is valuable as a preventive and also for women
recovering from breast cancer. In the latter case, it should be administered in consultation with your doctor or a professional nutritionist.

COLON POLYPS AND COLON CANCER

Every area in the world where people eat a diet high in animal fat
has a correspondingly high incidence of colon cancer. Indeed, the
more animal fat consumed, the more likely you are to get this
disease.

Given this fact, it is astonishing to me that anyone would opt for
a high-fat diet. In Japan, for example, where the population eats far
less meat and chicken than we do here, the incidence of colon cancer is far lower than ours, and lest you think this might have more
to do with genetics than diet, when Japanese move to this country
and adopt our diet, they get colon cancer with the same frequency
as the rest of us.

The reason that colon cancer and animal fats are linked is that
the fats lead to changes in the normal bacterial composition of the

intestine. The resulting abnormal bacteria can change harmless bile salts, produced by the gallbladder, into cancer-forming substances.

Fiber

The amount of time between eating food and eliminating its waste is called *transit time*. If transit time is lengthy, the waste sits too long in the colon, and the bowel wall is thereby exposed to potential carcinogenics for prolonged periods. In addition, excessive amounts of bowel toxins are absorbed into the blood.

Fiber is essential to moving waste through the blood. Fiber together with generous fluid intake (those 6 to 8 glasses of water a day) will make elimination regular and easy so that toxins do not build up, and your potential for colon cancer will markedly decrease. Meat, dairy products, and eggs contain no fiber. Neither do most processed foods. My Fourteen-Day Diet for lymphatic health, on the other hand, is high in fiber and in colon cancer–preventing micronutrients such as calcium and vitamin D.

Fiber and Polyps

Small growths on the colon, called polyps, can precede colon cancer. The condition is generally treated surgically, but research led by Dr. Jerome DeCasse while at the Medical College of Wisconsin showed that when 3,000 milligrams of vitamin C daily was given to over 3,000 patients with colon polyps, within six months over 50 percent of them reported a complete disappearance of the growths or a significant reduction.

Dr. DeCasse also studied the effect of fiber in the form of wheat bran on colon polyps. He discovered that if patients ate two bowls of All-Bran cereal daily, the polyps shrank.

All-Bran also has a dramatic effect on patients who have had malignant colon and rectal tumors surgically removed, by halting the early cell changes preceding a cancer recurrence in the remaining colon. Interestingly, wheat bran—as opposed to other fiber sources such as oats and corn—was the only food that halted these changes. All-Bran Buds are good tasting and deliver 13 grams of fiber in one-third cup.

Other foods that many be beneficial in preventing polyps are:

- Cold-water northern fish such as salmon, mackerel, sardines, and herring
- Cabbage and other cruciferous vegetables
- Pectin found in apples
- Yogurt containing *Lactobacillus acidophilus,* a normal bacterium abundant in a healthy bowel

If you have polyps, see your doctor, for only a physician can determine if cancer is present. And as a further preventive, avoid or reduce alcohol, especially beer.

A Vitamin and Mineral Plan for Colon Health, Colon Polyps, and Colon Cancer Prevention

High-potency multivitamin and mineral: VM 75 (Solgar), with iron for premenopausal women, without iron for men and postmenopausal women; 1 tablet daily

Calcium citrate plus magnesium (Twin Labs): 2 with breakfast, 2 with lunch, 4 at bedtime

Lactobacillus acidophilis: as directed on label

Max EPA fish oils: 1 g three times daily.

Vitamin C as calcium ascorbate: 1,000 mg three times daily.

Reminder: Unless specified, all vitamin and mineral supplements should be taken just before or after a meal.

A FINAL CHECKLIST: RECOMMENDATIONS FOR GETTING WELL FROM CANCER

1. Find a nutritionally aware physician in whom you have confidence to guide you in getting well.
2. Know that you *can* get well and that *you* play a large part in meeting this challenge.
3. Be positive and optimistic. There are survivors from every kind of cancer, including glioblastomas. Be one of them.
4. Take this shattering blow and turn it into a wake-up call that will affect the rest of your life for the better.
5. Read and listen to Dr. Bernie Siegel's books, tapes, and videos. *Practice* what he preaches.
6. Feed your mind what is good, true, and life-supporting. Make the most of every moment and every relationship.
7. Listen to a relaxation tape or music at least twice a day.
8. Immediately begin a health-supporting, organically grown, low-fat, high-fiber diet with supplements and with 6 to 8 glasses of water a day.
9. No caffeine. No alcohol. No smoking.

12

Asthma, Osteoarthritis, and Rheumatoid Arthritis

ASTHMA

Asthma is characterized by constriction and inflammation in the bronchial tubes that results in difficulty breathing, especially on exhalation. It is accompanied by coughing, shortness of breath, and a feeling of heaviness in the chest. Those who have suffered severe attacks describe it as like being in an airless tomb, producing abject terror. It is caused by one or a number of components, among them genetics, allergic sensitivities, and stress. An otherwise healthy woman I know had so pronounced an asthmatic reaction on being fired from her longtime job that she had to be rushed by ambulance to the hospital, and she was so sure she was going to die that her husband called me that evening to tell me she had no chance of surviving—only to call again the next day to announce that she was fine.

In 1990 there were 10 million cases of asthma, a 50 percent increase over 1980, and deaths have doubled in the last two decades. Asthma is most common in children under the age of ten (probably caused by poor diet, too many dairy products, and a lack of breast-feeding), and it afflicts twice as many boys as girls, for reasons we don't yet fully understand.

Treatment

Asthma is usually treated with drugs, avoidance of triggering agents and desensitization to them, and by stress-reduction techniques. Inhaled bronchodilators and inhaled steroids are now commonly used to treat chronic symptoms and as lifesaving medicines. However, natural methods exist for the treatment of asthma, that may lessen the need for such medications.

If at all possible, elimination of the cause is far better than battling symptoms. (When the bathtub is overflowing, do you turn off the faucets or continue to mop the floor?) In all disease, the greatest challenge is to search for the cause, find it, and eliminate it—and asthma is no exception.

One common cause is *diet*. One study showed that 92 percent of the patients observed with asthma improved significantly on a no-meat, no-dairy regimen. Garlic, onions, and hot and spicy foods such as mustard, horseradish, and hot chili peppers are beneficial for asthmatics, for they seem to act as nature's bronchodilators. Lots of vegetables and fruit are also helpful, probably due to their high vitamin C and bioflavonoid content. Thanks to its antihistamine effects, vitamin C reduces overall allergic sensitivities, and bioflavonoids produce similar effects.

Supplementation with vitamin C has been shown to reduce the number of asthma attacks. In one study, patients receiving 1 gram (1,000 milligrams) of vitamin C daily experienced a quarter as many attacks as those taking a placebo. In other studies, both asthmatic children and adults experienced a decrease in symptoms when taking a vitamin B_6 supplement. Vitamin E may be beneficial because of its antioxidant and anti-inflammatory properties. Intravenous magnesium has been used as an effective emergency treatment for acute attacks.

How to Deal with Triggering Agents

THE ENVIRONMENT
1. Take protective measures to avoid dust, mold, pets, and pollen, the common allergens.
2. Beware of chemicals in household products such as fabric softeners, cleaners, and new carpeting.
3. Do not smoke.
4. Minimize exposure to cold air, which is a common asthma trigger. When outside in the winter, breathe through your nose and use a scarf over your mouth, if necessary.
5. Avoid woodstoves and fireplaces.
6. Avoid air pollution if possible, especially when exercising.
7. Install air filters in your home and office.

STRESS As I've noted earlier, there are stresses you can avoid, others you cannot. But even in a high-powered job or during a tricky period at home, you can learn relaxation responses, pay attention to your breathing, get as much rest as possible, and learn to think positively. Self-hypnosis and biofeedback have proved beneficial in reducing the symptoms and frequency of asthma attacks.

DIET Asthmatics are 300 percent more likely to have food allergies than nonasthmatics. Common offenders are:

Additives and preservatives

Eggs

Chocolate

Margarine

Citrus fruits

Nuts

Coconut, corn, palm, and
    peanut oils

Shellfish

Soy

Corn

Sugar

Dairy products

Wheat

Avoid soft drinks, MSG, food colorings (especially yellow dye #5), and preservatives such as BHA. Sulfates are often added to processed foods: read the labels. They can be unsuspected in restaurant food, mainly in fruits, vegetables, salads, and especially in avocado dip. Test strips are available to detect their presence, and you should use them if your asthma is connected to food allergies. Beware of "hidden" nuts, particularly peanuts, used in many food oils. Some asthmatics may be sensitive to aspirin and to nonsteroidal anti-inflammatory drugs such as ibuprofen.

"Good" foods include freshwater salmon, herring, freshwater tuna, mackerel, and sardines, eaten three times weekly. Taking fresh fish-oil capsules may help. Green tea is vital. Omega-3 fatty acids should be stressed. And my Fourteen-Day Diet for lymphatic health, modified along the lines described above, should be your standard diet.

A Vitamin and Mineral Plan for Asthma

Note: All dosages are for adults and should be used only under the guidance of your doctor. Check all vitamin, mineral, and herbal preparations for possible food allergens.

High-potency multivitamin and mineral: VM 75 (Solgar), with iron for premenopausal women, without iron for men and postmenopausal women; 1 tablet daily

Vitamin C as ascorbic acid, calcium ascorbate, or ester C: 1 g 3 times daily

Vitamin E: 400 IU daily. In the presence of hypertension, diabetes, or rheumatic heart disease, begin with 100 IU daily and increase to 400 IU daily over six weeks.

B_{12}: shots if possible. 1 mg daily for 2 weeks to see if helpful. If injections are unavailable, take sublingual B_{12} tablets, 1 to 3 mg daily.

Magnesium citrate: 400 mg daily. Magnesium occasionally may cause diarrhea. If so, lower dosage to half.

Calcium citrate plus magnesium (Twin Labs): 4 at bedtime

Folic acid: 400 mcg daily

Selenium: 200 mcg taken with vitamin E daily

Herbs: Licorice, ginko biloba—as directed on label or by health-care professional

Fish oils: 3 gms daily. Can thin the blood and interact with warfarin.

Reminder: Unless specified, all vitamin and mineral supplements should be taken just before or after a meal.

OSTEOARTHRITIS

Osteoarthritis is a degenerative disease of the joints, a crippling condition that plagues 40 million Americans, 80 percent of them over the age of fifty. The joints crack and creak when moved, and there is local soreness and sometimes swelling. Other symptoms may include stiffness in the morning and pain in the use of the joint, which can be relieved by rest. Generally affected are the weight-bearing joints of the body—knees, hips, and spine. The joints of the hands are also vulnerable.

Osteoarthritis often makes its appearance subtly, generally starting with stiff fingers on awakening. The process of the disease involves the breakdown of cartilage and other tissues that enable the joints to move freely. This form of arthritis is characterized by pain and swelling but none of the inflammation and joint deformity of rheumatoid arthritis. It is seen as a natural process of aging, but joint injury can play a part, and so can genetics; clearly, some people are more prone to it than others.

Treatment

Aspirin is the most common drug used to fight the disease, but since it must be taken in high doses, there is a danger of bleeding in the stomach lining. Ear ringing, or tinnitus, is also associated with aspirin toxicity.

The nonsteroidal anti-inflammatory drugs such as ibuprofen were expected to relieve pain and inflammation just as aspirin does but without aspirin's side effects. However, they have their own side effects, including the danger of stomach ulcers, severe gastrointestinal bleeding, and kidney and liver damage. Also, although the drugs may alleviate the pain and swelling temporarily, they may actually accelerate cartilage destruction by hiding the symptoms and speeding up the progression of the disease.

The idea that arthritis may be related to what we eat is not a new one. Some people seem sensitive to a group of vegetables known as the "nightshades"—tomatoes, white potatoes, green peppers, eggplant. Other foods that may cause arthritis pain include wheat and dairy products.

There is no question that the heavier you are, the more the stress load on your joints, so my Fourteen-Day Diet for lymphatic health, which normalizes weight, or any one of a variety of weight-loss diets is strongly advised. Fish oils may be beneficial in treating inflammation—eating cold-water fish such as salmon, tuna, mackerel, or sardines (or fish oil capsules as a supplement) may be helpful. Avoid margarine, corn oil, peanut oil, coconut oil, and palm oil, all of which may encourage inflammation.

Among the vitamins, C and E appear to enhance the stability of joint cartilage and are essential for the repair of connective tissue. Glucosamine sulfate is a major component of the cartilage itself, which diminishes as we age. It appears to be an effective treatment for osteoarthritis, and though it may take longer to work than the anti-inflammatory drugs and painkillers, it does not have their side effects.

Exercise is essential to keep muscles strong and joints moving. Swimming is often preferred because the joints are free to move without having to bear weight. Physical therapy with massage, heat, cold, and ultrasound, in conjunction with exercise, often helps to improve specific joint mobility and to reduce joint pain. Yoga for relaxation and stress reduction, stretching, and acupuncture may all alleviate symptoms. And some patients have discovered remarkable effects with magnet therapy.

A Vitamin and Mineral Plan for Osteoarthritis

High-potency multivitamin and mineral: VM 75 (Solgar), with iron for premenopausal women, without iron for men and postmenopausal women; 1 tablet daily

Vitamin C as calcium ascorbate or ester C: 1,000 mg three times daily

Calcium citrate plus magnesium (Twin Labs): 2 with breakfast, 2 with lunch, 4 at bedtime

Cod-liver oil: 1 tablespoon daily with juice as per instructions, along with two 8-ounce glasses of water with *Green Magma.* When taking cod-liver oil for an extended time (over three weeks), discontinue multiple vitamin (excess vitamin A and D over time may be toxic).

Flaxseed oil: 1 tablespoon daily. Keep refrigerated.

Glucosamine chondroitin formula (Country Life): 1 capsule 3 times daily

Selenium: 200 mcg daily

Boron: 3 mg daily

Zinc: 20 mg daily. Check your multivitamin to see if it contains zinc. Do not exceed 30 mg.

Vitamin B$_6$: 60 mg daily

Vitamin E: 400 IU daily. In the presence of hypertension, diabetes, or rheumatic heart disease, begin with 100 IU daily and increase to 400 IU daily over six weeks.

Later if needed: *Vitamin B$_3$* (niacinamide): 800 mg twice daily. Warning: High doses can temporarily cause liver irritation. Medical supervision is advised. Especially effective with knee problems.

BOTANICALS

Bilberry: up to 80 mg in capsules three times daily

Boswellin: as directed on label

Hawthorn berry: as directed on label

MSM: 500 mg twice daily. Can be increased to 1,000 mg twice daily.

SAMe (S-adenosylmethimine): 200 mg twice daily for the first two days, increase to 400 mg twice daily on day 3, then to 400 mg three times daily on day 10. After twenty-one days at a dosage of 1,200 mg daily, reduce dosage to the maintenance level of 200 mg twice daily. (This is an expensive supplement.)

Sea cucumber extract: as directed on label

Reminder: Unless specified, all vitamin and mineral supplements should be taken just before or after a meal.

RHEUMATOID ARTHRITIS

Unlike osteoarthritis, rheumatoid arthritis affects the whole body. It is an autoimmune disease; that is, the immune system, usually able to protect the body from invaders, actually attacks its own tissue—the lining of the joints. The most frequently involved joints are the wrists, hands, feet, and the spine in the neck region. It starts with vague joint pain and stiffness, then develops into swollen, damaged joints and can be debilitating, even crippling. Rheumatoid arthritis can affect the lungs, intestines, vascular system, skin, and nervous system. It can cause fever, weight loss, and severe fatigue. Some patients with the disease improve; others suffer rapid joint destruction and severe disabilities.

Here too, aspirin and nonsteroidal anti-inflammatory drugs are used, but again there is a danger of unwelcome side effects. Steroids have been shown to be effective, but they often have a host of side effects; and other medicines, including gold, antimalarial drugs, and a chemotherapy drug used for cancer called methotrexate, which are sometimes prescribed, have the potential for serious toxicity. In the most severe cases, surgery and joint replacement are performed. In no case should you attempt self-medication. Rheumatoid arthritis can be extremely serious, and any battle against it must be undertaken with a doctor as your ally.

Diet has been strongly implicated in both the cause and cure of rheumatoid arthritis. Studies have shown that in societies where a more "primitive" diet (such as roots and vegetables) is eaten, rheumatoid arthritis is virtually nonexistent, whereas a high rate of the disease is found in countries like ours that consume the typical Western diet.

My Fourteen-Day Diet for lymphatic health appears to protect against the disease, yet food allergies and sensitivities have been shown in some people to play a major role in its onslaught, so be careful even if you follow my plan. The most common foods that can aggravate the disease are wheat, corn, milk, the nightshade vegetables (tomatoes, potatoes, eggplant, peppers), and food additives. Certain fats, such as butter, margarine, fried foods, and the so-called saturated or hydrogenated fats may increase inflammation, and oils such as corn, peanut, coconut, and palm are likewise harmful. On the other hand, "good" fats—the omega-3 fatty acids—may act to prevent inflammation. Cold-water northern fish—cod, salmon, tuna, sardines, and mackerel—are, as we've seen, rich in these fats.

Certain foods and spices possess antioxidants that can also help limit the inflammation by protecting the joint tissues from deterioration. Of particular benefit are fresh fruits and vegetables, especially dark red and blue berries such as blueberries and cherries. Ginger and the active ingredient in curry powder called curcumin also reduce inflammation.

Stress can have a particularly negative effect on the body and thus trigger and worsen symptoms. Yoga, biofeedback, meditation, and massage are effective means of reducing stress levels, and exercise is also important, swimming in particular. All are restorative to mental and physical power.

A Vitamin and Mineral Plan for Rheumatoid Arthritis

High-potency multivitamin and mineral: VM 75 (Solgar), with iron for premenopausal women, without iron for men and postmenopausal women; 1 tablet daily

Vitamin C as calcium ascorbate or ester C: 1,000 mg three times daily

Vitamin E: 400 IU daily. In the presence of hypertension, diabetes, or rheumatic heart disease, begin with 100 IU daily and increase to 400 IU daily over six weeks

Mixed carotenes: as directed on label

Calcium citrate plus magnesium (Twin Labs): 2 with breakfast, 2 with lunch, 4 at bedtime

Copper: 2 mg daily

Selenium: 200 mcg daily

Manganese: 10 mg daily

Zinc: 20 mg daily. Check your multivitamin to see if it contains zinc. Do not exceed 30 mg.

Bromelain: 500 mg three times daily between meals for a trial of at least three weeks

Ginger: 500 mg three times daily

Max EPA fish oils: 3 to 5 g daily. Much higher doses have been used with rheumatoid arthritis, but only under a doctor's supervision.

Glucosamine chondroitin formula (Country Life): 1 capsule 3 times daily

Reminder: Unless specified, all vitamin and mineral supplements should be taken just before or after a meal.

13

Aging

It seems appropriate to end a book on health with a few thoughts on aging.

Aging is not a disease; indeed, it can be a blessing. Yet in Western cultures, and particularly in America, it is considered a condition to be avoided. Here we are told to fight against the "aging process." Our television ads (and television sitcoms) are mainly aimed at the young, and we are infected with the mind-set that being thirty-something is already a long way toward the grave. To us, aging is, as Stephan Rechtschaffen writes, "an anathema. It's as though every new wrinkle requires a smoothing cream, every grey hair a dye, every aching joint a liniment. We run from aging, we deny it, and we are embarrassed by it."

In other societies, and particularly in the East, old age is known as a time of wisdom, of tranquillity, of contemplation and spirituality. The elderly are honored, not avoided; listened to, admired, seen as the purveyors of knowledge. The knowledge they impart is not necessarily about facts but about the emotional and instinctual sides of our beings. They've "been there, done that," and they can teach us life lessons if only we pay them heed.

THE BIOLOGY OF AGING

We don't want to age, yet we do everything in our power to live longer. We know that life is a process having both quantity and quality, but even if the quality is poor, either physically or emotionally, we usually wish to prolong it (and this is true for all cultures), for the alternative means an end to existence in this world, and who knows what may lie beyond? What we want is to live into old age productively, to avoid deterioration as much as possible, to maintain agility and mental acuity, to be, as a friend of mine's mother is, a "young ninety-five."

Thus the scientific community has studied the aging process intensely. The questions of why cells stop multiplying (although it has recently been discovered that brain cells, at least, regenerate as we age), why bones become brittle, why hair grays, and why memory fails have come under intense scrutiny, and particularly in the last three decades, new evidence has come to light.

In the early 1970s, it was postulated that free radicals and oxidative stress were the cause not only of chronic degenerative diseases but of aging itself. Subsequent research has validated this theory and has demonstrated that oxidation of lipids and mutation and breakdown of the DNA that produces enzymes and messengers are important parts of the aging process. It stands to reason, then, that if we avoid strong oxidative processes like radiation and smog, and if we follow a good diet and exercise program (it's never too late to start, although if we start early our chances are better), we can extend the functional age of our bodies and minds.

Further scientific investigation evaluated the phenomenon of *apoptosis*—programmed cell death—which is a winding down of the cell's function so that it fails to metabolize and simply dies. Microscopic examination of an apoptotic cell shows an essentially normal-looking cell that has one drawback: it no longer functions. The present theory is that at some point the DNA in the cell sends it a message that it should shut down its metabolic (energy) plants in the mitochondria and not reproduce anymore—in effect, closing itself down. As noted, this process can be hastened by oxidative stress, though it is eventually inevitable.

Another important factor in the aging process is *glycation,* which is the caramelization or burning of the glycoproteins in our body. Glycoproteins are chemical compounds made of sugar and proteins that are an integral part of our tissue. When oxidative stress occurs and attacks the sugar radical of the glycoprotein, the sugar becomes caramelized, the way that heating sugar for a prolonged period makes caramel. (Brown sugar is oxidized sucrose.) When glycation takes place, the glycoprotein loses its integrity and becomes useless in hormonal reactions. Age spots and brown spots are a good example of this "caramelization" in the skin.

The last area of importance for aging under the heading of oxidative stress is the production of *metalloprotease,* enzymes that break down the proteins in collagen and elastin. These are released in inflammatory reactions or oxidative stress situations. When they are released, they break the collagen bonds and the elastic membrane layer that maintains the integrity of certain tissues like the arteries and the skin, thereby creating sagging and wrinkles.

SLOWING AGING

The single unifying factor in all these processes is oxidative stress, which is why I say that if you minimize it, you can slow the aging process. Besides the standard principles for antioxidation, aging can be approached with the Lemole formula of decreasing the toxic load, reinforcing the antioxidative defenses, and improving the lymphatic flow to clear the body of toxins and inflammatory by-products.

A diet of complex carbohydrates, low in fat and protein and avoiding simple sugars like sucrose, glucose, and fructose, will delay oxidative stress and prevent glycation. Besides the usual antioxidants found in my Fourteen-Day Diet for lymphatic health, I'd add 500 milligrams of alpha lipoic acid three times a day. It has the unusual advantage of being both lipid- and fat-soluble, so it can concentrate not only in the cell membrane but also in the fluid— the cytosol—of the cell. It can permeate the cytosol and bathe the DNA to prevent mutation of the DNA and the migration of inflammatory messengers, from proinflammatory proteins produced by the DNA in the center of the cell, to the cell membrane and then to the body.

Other supplements useful to stem the aging process are para-aminobenzoic acid (PABA), an amino acid beneficial in preserving the elasticity of the skin, and pantothene, recommended for healthy hair and preventing gray hair and baldness.

OTHER AGING PROBLEMS AND THEIR TREATMENT

Bone shrinking is a sign of aging. It not only causes osteoporosis and back deformity but also changes the appearance of the face in that the jaw and cheekbones recede, causing the facial tissue to sag and the teeth to become loose in their sockets. Exercise will slow shrinkage by increasing cardiovascular and muscle tone and normalize the bone architecture by preserving calcium and magnesium.

Another problem is the loss of water in the skin. Keeping water in with salves and creams helps this condition, as does living in a not-too-dry atmosphere. Avoiding sunlight also prevents the skin from drying out and causing wrinkles and protects against skin cancers like melanoma and squamous cell carcinoma. Smoking causes small artery spasms in the skin, which in turn lead to the death of the muscles underneath the skin, meaning that scar tissue is deposited beneath the surface of your face—the cause of wrinkles. I've often thought that perhaps a better way to stop young girls from smoking (and they are the fastest-growing portion of the smoking population) is to tell them not that they'll develop cancer but that they'll age prematurely.

If you want to avoid the dark rings under your eyes that often come with age, give up coffee and alcohol. And the sour look that sometimes accompanies old age may not come from bitterness at the aging process but rather from a magnesium deficiency that usually accelerates as we get older: 400 to 1,200 milligrams of magnesium a day will give a glow to your face.

AGING "TREATMENT"

- Make sure you eat a diet high in complex carbohydrates, including vegetables and fruits and featuring monounsaturated and polyunsaturated oils (the Fourteen-Day Diet for lymphatic health is ideal).
- Avoid animal fats, coconut fats, trans-fats, hydrogenated oil, and shortening. A diet high in saturated fats has been linked to dry skin.
- Make sure your diet contains omega-3 fatty acids, including walnut oil, fish oils, pumpkin, sunflower, and sesame seeds.
- Add supplements (see pages 207 to 209): folic acid, vita-

min E, selenium, essential fatty acids, lecithin, vitamin A, zinc, aloe vera, and jojoba oil (as directed).

- Use a good skin moisturizer daily.
- Avoid overexposure to the sun and tanning booths. When you must go out, especially in the midday sun, be sure to wear a hat and sunglasses.
- Use mild soaps and cleansers.
- Buy a humidifier for your home.
- Exercise regularly to increase blood and lymph circulation and oxygen intake. (The young ninety-five-year-old woman I mentioned previously walks 1 mile a day and exercises with 2-pound weights for ten minutes three times a week for upper-body strength.)
- If you haven't already, institute a program of regular massage.
- Practice relaxation techniques such as yoga.
- Meditate.
- Maintain an optimistic outlook. Mental attitude is very important in keeping us young, not only in the production of (positive) endorphins and enkephalins but in eliminating the (negative) release of hormones that accelerate oxidative stress. Constant frowning or scowling leaves permanent traces on the skin, which then become the creases characteristic of age. Remember: It takes four times as many muscles to frown as it does to smile.
- Follow a regular spiritual practice.

The regimen for aging, then, is much like the one I recommend for all ages. The river of life can flow smoothly and for many decades in each of us. But we cannot take it for granted. It is up to us to make sure it keeps flowing.

Index

Page numbers in *italics* refer to illustrations.